Health Promotion, Disease Prevention, and Exercise Epidemiology

Nellie M. Cyr

University Press of America,® Inc.

Dallas · Lanham · Boulder · New York · Oxford

Copyright © 2003 by
University Press of America,® Inc.
4501 Forbes Boulevard
Suite 200
Lanham, Maryland 20706
UPA Acquisitions Department (301) 459-3366

PO Box 317
Oxford
OX2 9RU, UK

Library of Congress Control Number: 2003111461
ISBN 0-7618-2716-1 (paperback : alk. ppr.)

⊖™ The paper used in this publication meets the minimum
requirements of American National Standard for Information
Sciences—Permanence of Paper for Printed Library Materials,
ANSI Z39.48—1984

- TO MY HUSBAND, DAVE

TABLE OF CONTENTS

PREFACE

There are many positive aspects to an advanced technological society. Remote controls to change the television channel and open the garage door are very prevalent in our society. Machines that blow the snow and throw the leaves have replaced shoveling the snow and raking the leaves. Electric hedge clippers, weed-whackers, and other yard amenities have replaced manually operated devices. Golfers can choose to sit comfortably in an electric cart instead of walking a few miles around the golf course. High-tech appliances have made housework physically less demanding, and drive-through banks and fast food restaurants have made daily chores less cumbersome.

As is true with most things in life, for every upside there exists a downside. Our advanced technological society has made life more comfortable and more enjoyable, but it has also resulted in less movement, less activity, and an overall under active society. Concurrently, Americans are getting fatter. Factors that contribute to the increased prevalence of obesity include an increased portion size combined with the early childhood lesson to "finish everything on your plate", and the abundant availability of appealing and relatively inexpensive food. Consequentially, we have become a society that consumes more calories than we expend.

Research has indicated that two out of every three Americans do not get enough exercise, and one out of every four do not exercise at all. The physiological consequences of inactivity are evident in the increased prevalence of chronic diseases including type 2 diabetes, hypertension, obesity, and subsequently cardiovascular disease; this nation's number one cause of death. This textbook explores the physiological mechanisms and consequences of an under active society.

Excessive body fat, and obesity are critical public health issues as 61% of all Americans are either overweight or obese. The World Health Organization, and the National Heart, Lung, and Blood

Institute have classified obesity as an epidemic. Since 1960, the overall prevalence of obesity has doubled. This dramatic increase is evident in all subgroups of the American population, particularly among children and young adults, where the rates have tripled. The consequence of this trend is the evident dramatic increases in the incidence of type 2 diabetes in our society, particularly within younger age groups. This textbook explores and explains the relationship between obesity and cardiovascular disease.

Research has demonstrated that daily behavioral choices contribute to over 50% of an individual's health. Individual choices to exercise or to not be active, to eat healthy meals or choose foods high in saturated fat, and whether to smoke or abstain are strong determinants of overall health.

This book explores the concept of prevention in the form of health promotion programs. Substantial research studies are referenced, and extensive data analysis is provided to substantiate the concept of prevention. Physical activity serves as the base in the foundation of prevention and is supported by cumulative epidemiological evidence. Complex biological, biochemical, and physiological mechanisms of exercise, and chronic disease are explained, and are correlated to improved physiological health.

Public health officials have long contented that a small increase in activity among the least active segment of our population could dramatically improve health and decrease cardiovascular disease risk factors, subsequently lowing cardiovascular disease rates. The research analysis and statistical data presented in this textbook supports this theory and confirms the need to focus public health efforts towards the least active segments of our population.

Prevention is the key to reducing cardiovascular disease and the chronic diseases that permeate our society. Participation in daily physical activity, and learning to adopt daily lifestyle choices that have a positive impact on personal health are cornerstones to a healthy society.

~ Nellie M. Cyr, Ph.D.

ACKNOWLEDGEMENTS

An endeavor such as this could not be accomplished without the support of many people. I would like to thank my family and friends for their encouragement as well as the individuals who provided research assistance. Special thanks to Carmen Cyr Bailey for her help with typesetting, William Collins for his editorial expertise, and David Cyr for his graphic wizardry.

CHAPTER ONE

HEALTH PROMOTION AND CARDIOVASCULAR DISEASE

This chapter provides the rationale and establishes the foundation for prevention. It introduces the concept of health promotion and disease prevention and discusses the risk factors associated with cardiovascular disease.

The escalating cost of health care is slowly outpacing society's ability to pay for it. In 1960, national health expenditures consumed 5.1% of the Gross Domestic Product (GDP) or $27 billion. In 1985, the numbers grew to 10.1 % of the GDP, or $430 billion. In the year 2003, the cost rose to 15.2% of the GDP, as Americans spent $1.66 trillion on health care. Government projections estimate that health care costs will increase about 7% annually though the next decade as the cost of hospital services and prescription drugs continue to increase. Projections for health care expenditures from 2008-2012 predict that consumers will spend $2.4 trillion in 2008, $3 trillion in 2010, and $3.1 trillion, or 17.7% of the GDP by 2012, and an astonishing $13 trillion, or 26% of GDP, by 2030 (Figure 1.1).[1,2] With an average expenditure of about $5,000.00 per citizen,

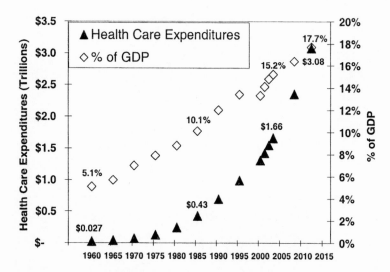

FIGURE 1.1 - Annual health care expenditures and health care expenditures as a percent of Gross Domestic Product (GDP), 1960-2015. *Source:* Trends in U.S. Health Care Spending, 2001 [Electronic Version]. Health Accounts, Volume 22:1. Centers for Medicare and Medicaid Services. http://cms.hhs.gov/statistics/nhe/default.asp. April, 2003.

Americans spend more money on health care than any other country in the world.[3] Proposed reasons for the substantial cost of health care include:

- Advances in medical research and state-of-the-art technology
- Demographics – the fact that Americans are living longer, thereby requiring more medical intervention
- The expectation that individuals can receive the best care necessitates excellent educational and training facilities
- The organization of the third party payer system
- Medical malpractice insurance premiums

The organizations responsible for paying health care bills include public entities: federal and state governments, and private groups: insurance companies, and corporate employers. As the costs continue to escalate, the government and private insurance providers have had to increase their contribution to the cost. American corporations contributed 18% of the estimated cost in 1965, 25% of the costs in 1985, 28% in 1991, and 30% in 1997, which resulted in a decreased profit margin. Estimates have concluded that over 50% of business profits are spent on employee and dependent health care.[4-6]

While cost-containment represents a major concern to business leaders, a secondary, less recognized factor is the actual allocation of health care resources. It has been estimated that 88% of all costs related to health care are allocated towards primary care (medical care services or products), and less than 2% of the resources are allocated towards health promotion or primary prevention.[5] This, despite the evidence that lifestyle choices, which have been estimated to contribute to over 50% of an individual's health, are strongly correlated to the leading causes of death and disability in the United States.[7]

Chronic disease accounts for approximately 75% of health care costs each year.[3] The number one contributor to health care costs and the leading chronic disease contributor to premature morbidity and mortality in the nation is cardiovascular disease (CVD).[8] In 1990, the estimated cost of CVD was $135 billion.[9] In 2003, it was expected to reach $209 billion, an increase of 55 %.[3] In 2003, the cost of heart disease and stroke, including health care expenditures and lost productivity from death and disability, was estimated at $351 billion.

Epidemiological evidence has suggested that the incidence of cardiovascular disease can be significantly reduced by an increase in physical activity.[10-13] Research studies have demonstrated that a sedentary person runs almost twice the risk of developing heart disease than the most active person.[13] Research studies have also demonstrated that habitual exercisers have lower blood pressure,[14-15] improved lipid profiles,[15-16] and increased cardiovascular fitness values.[15-17] Physical activity has also been shown to modify cardiovascular disease risk factors such as hypertension, obesity, and undesirable blood lipid profiles.[13,18]

CVD risk factors have traditionally been divided into groups, major or minor, and as modifiable or unmodifiable. Included among major modifiable risk factors are hypertension, obesity, type 2 diabetes, inactivity, hyperlipidemia, and cigarette smoking. In 1995, hypertension was evident in 50 million people or 20% of the U.S. population.[14] Today, 28% of adults have high blood pressure, while an additional 30 million have high-normal blood pressure.[19] New language has been instituted to describe any blood pressure value that falls between 120/80 mmHg, and 140/90 mmHg. The new descriptor, which affects 45 million Americans, is pre-hypertension, and it denotes the significance of an increased blood pressure value and its relationship to hypertension. Hypertension is associated with higher cardiovascular morbidity and mortality rates.[20] Causative factors include obesity, high sodium intake, excessive consumption of alcohol, and physical inactivity. While the hemodynamic mechanism is not clear, physically active individuals have lower blood pressure than do sedentary persons. Two large epidemiological studies have shown that people with hypertension that were physically active had a 40-60% lower mortality rate than did otherwise comparable unfit and sedentary hypertensives.[14] Physical activity, along with four other nonpharmacological modalities, is currently employed to reduce arterial pressure: dietary sodium restriction, moderation of alcohol intake, smoking cessation, and weight control.[20]

Overweight has been defined as a body mass index (BMI) of between 25-29.9, and obesity has been defined as a BMI of greater than 30. Comparing world-wide data, Americans have a greater percentage of people classified as obese than almost any other country in the world.[21] Sixty-one percent of Americans, including 35% of college students have a BMI of greater than 25, which means that more than six out of every ten of Americans are categorized as having too much fat. In 1980, 14.5% of Americans were obese as compared with 26% in 1999. Since 1960, the prevalence of obesity has almost doubled, and over the last ten years, the average adult has gained an average of eight pounds. Overweight and obesity are now the second leading causes of preventable death in the USA, and cost about $61 billion in direct medical costs.[3]

Obesity predisposes an individual to hypertension, diabetes, hypercholesterolemia, and is an independent risk factor for coronary heart disease and stroke.[22-23] Nonpharmacological intervention strategies to reduce percent body fat include decreasing dietary fat intake to <30% of total calories, reducing saturated fats to <10% of total calories, and increasing physical activity. Recent research has reported a positive correlation between moderate-intensity activities and weight loss, and a corresponding improvement in cardiovascular disease risk factors.[15,24-27]

Epidemiological evidence suggests that a causal relationship exists between elevated plasma lipid levels and both the development and progression of coronary heart disease (CHD) (Figure 1.2). Decreasing both total serum cholesterol levels and low-

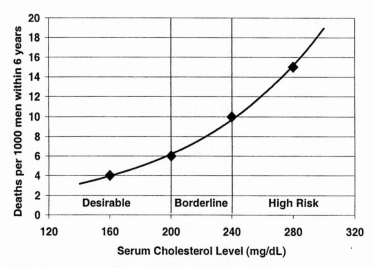

FIGURE 1.2 - Deaths per 1000 men within 6 years at various levels of serum cholesterol. *Source:* Lauer, MS, Fontanrosa, PB. Updated Guidelines of Cholesterol Management. *JAMA* 2001;285:2508.

density lipoproteins (LDL) lowers the risk for CHD, while an inverse relationship exists between circulating high density lipoproteins (HDL) and CHD risk (Figure 1.3).[28]

While the mechanism is not clear, exercise has been shown to improve serum lipid levels, perhaps by increasing the activity of lipoprotein lipase (LPL), and altering the activity of hepatic lipase (HP) and lecithin-cholesterol acyltransferase (LCAT), important enzymes in cholesterol metabolism.[29]

Tobacco use is responsible for more than one of every six deaths in the United States and is the single most preventable cause of death and disability in our society.[30] Direct medical expenditures attributed to smoking total more than $75 billion annually.[3] Cigarette smoking has consistently been associated with higher rates of stroke, peripheral vascular disease, and sudden cardiac death.[30]

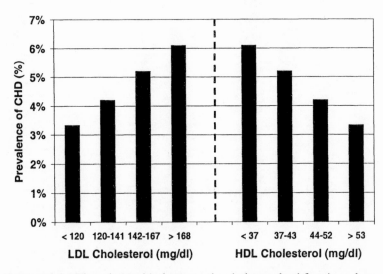

FIGURE 1.3 - The relationship between the cholesterol subfractions, low density lipoprotein [LDL], high density lipoproteins [HDL], and the prevalence of CHD. *Source:* McArdle, W D, Katch, FI, & Katch, V L. *Exercise Physiology: Energy, Nutrition and Human Performance (5th ed.).* p. 898. Boston: Lippincott, Williams and Wilkins, 2001.

Referring to the consequences of smoking specific to the cardiovascular system, Becker states, "multiple physiological mechanisms acting synergistically cause endothelial injury, an abnormal intravascular environment and abnormalities in both the electrical conducting system and the function of ventricular myocardium."[31] Smoking cessation has been associated with reduced cardiovascular complications to the extent that it has been recognized as being more effective at reducing mortality in the aggregate of smokers with known coronary heart disease than beta-blocker therapy, coronary bypass surgery (CABG) or coronary angioplasty (PCTA).[32]

While physical inactivity has been associated with hypertension, obesity and hyperlipidemia, physical activity has been associated with a decrease in coronary artery disease. Paffenberger investigated the relationship between physical activity and the attributable death rate due to coronary artery disease (CAD) in longshoremen and found that men with less active jobs sustained higher CAD death rates.[33] Cumulative epidemiological evidence has led groups such as the American Heart Association and the U.S. Public Health Service to proclaim physical inactivity as a risk factor for the development of cardiovascular disease and to classify it as a major public health concern that requires attention.[15,34-36]

Corporate leaders, in response to higher health care costs, have taken the initiative to develop strategies to reduce costs, including the initiation of programs to reduce the need for medical services. These preventive or health promotion programs have grown over the past 18 years. In 1985, 46% of 5,000 CEO's of the largest firms reported that their firms were sponsoring wellness/disease prevention programs. Thirty-eight percent indicated they had plans to initiate or were considering the adoption of these programs.[37] By 1988, almost two-thirds (65.8%) of all companies with more than 50 employees offered some type of wellness or health promotion activities.[38] It was estimated that by 1995 over one-half of America's largest corporations would offer comprehensive health promotion programs.[39] Three years later, in 1998, the reported percentage of companies with comprehensive health promotion programs was

55%.[40] While these percentages fell short of the Healthy People 2000 goal of 85%, the increase in comprehensive employee based health promotion programs has been encouraging. Early research on the financial efficacy of health promotion programs revealed inconsistencies in the employer's ability to quantify monetary benefits.[41] In 1995, a meta-analysis on the cost-effectiveness of health promotion programs proved to be revealing.[42] In this review, the authors analyzed 25 studies utilizing eight parameters as selection criteria. Each criterion measurement was defined in the publication. To be included in the analysis, each health promotion program had to include the following variables:

(a) at least three interventions (e.g., stress management, fitness, blood lipids);
(b) employer sponsored programs;
(c) quasi-experimental or true experimental studies;
(d) original results;
(e) economic variables had to be analyzed (calculations of benefits);
(f) the study had to be published in a peer review journal;
(g) the study had to utilize a control or comparison group; and,
(h) the author(s) must have employed statistical analysis.

After extensive analysis, the authors derived an average cost-benefit ratio of 1:5.94, with a range of 1:2.05 to 1:19.4. Restated, for every dollar an employer invested in a health promotion program, the net savings was almost six dollars (Figure 1.4).

More recently, between 1995-2003, additional published studies have substantiated the early research on financial efficacy, and additional researchers have been able to quantify monetary benefits from the implementation of health promotion programs.[40] As reported in Forbes Magazine, Johnson & Johnson, a leader in health promotion programs, saved $13 million a year in absenteeism

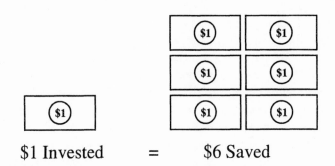

$1 Invested   = $6 Saved

FIGURE 1.4 - Return on investment. One dollar invested in health promotion programs results in six dollars saved.

and health care costs. Union Pacific saved an estimated $3 million per year by reducing hypertension and smoking among its employees. The most recent published meta-analysis found a wide range of return on investment estimates, from a low of $1.50 in benefits, or savings per dollar spent, to a high of $13.00 in benefits or savings per dollar spent.[43] The authors conclude that the wide savings range can be attributed to the variety of programs and services offered to the multitude of investigations and methodologies employed during the analysis.

Perhaps more important than the financial efficacy of preventive programs is the shift in the emphasis of health promotion programs from a focus on productivity to an improvement of health, with more altruistic companies viewing this as a beneficial social goal in itself. Initial research studies on the physiological benefits of health promotion programs have provided a foundation to build the argument for the appropriation of resources for preventive programs. In a case-control study, Shi examined the effects of an employee fitness program on selected physiological parameters and concluded that individuals who were exposed to fitness classes of varying intensities and duration experienced gains in maximal oxygen uptake (VO_2 max), flexibility, and a decrease in percent body fat.[44] Additional research studies in the 1990's supported Shi's findings. More recent research has corroborated earlier work on the physiological benefits of physical activity and the subsequent reduction in cardiovascular disease risk.[10-11,15,25-27,45-50] While numerous studies have laid a foundation, additional research is necessary to continue to substantiate the argument that prevention is more proactive, cost-effective, and socially redeeming than conventional medical treatment. As employers continue to examine both the cost-effectiveness and the social efficacy of these programs, further documentation is necessary to continue to strengthen the relationship between health promotion programs, decreased cardiovascular disease, and improved employee health.

REFERENCES

1. Centers for Medicare and Medicaid Services. *Health Accounts.* [http://cms.hhs.gov/statistics/nhe/default.asp]. April, 2003.

2. Letsch, S.W., Lazenby, H.C., Levit, K.R., & Cowan, C. (1994). "American National Health Expenditures." In P.R. Lee & L.L. Estes (Eds.), *The Nation's Health.* (4th ed., pp. 252-262). Boston: Jones and Bartlett.

3. Centers for Disease Control and Prevention. *The Promise of Prevention. Reducing the Health and Economic Burden of Chronic Disease.* Atlanta: Department of Health and Human Services, Centers for Disease Control and Prevention, February, 2003.

4. Everly, G.S., & Feldman, R.H. (Eds.). (1985). *Occupational Health Promotion: Health Behavior in the Workplace.* New York: John Wiley and Sons.

5. Ware, B. (1982). "Health education in occupational settings: History has its message." *Health Education Quarterly* 9 (supp), 37-41.

6. Chenoweth, D.H. (1998). *Worksite Health Promotion.* (p. 3). New Bern, NC: Human Kinetics.

7. Elsenrath, D. Hettler, B., Leafgren, F. (1988). Lifestyle Assessment Questionnaire (8th ed.), University of Wisconsin, Stevens Point, National Wellness Institute.

8. Cerny, F.J. (2001). *Exercise Physiology for Health Care Professionals.* (p. 233). Illinois: Human Kinetics.

9. U.S. Department of Health and Human Services. (1990). *Healthy People 2000 National Health Promotion and Disease Prevention Objectives.* (DHHS Publication No PHS 91-50213). Washington, DC: Government Printing Office (5)392-395.

10. Blair, S. (1996). "Physical inactivity and cardiovascular disease risk in women." *Medicine and Science in Sports and Exercise* 28, 9-10.

11. Blair, S. (1995). "Effects of physical activity on cardiovascular disease mortality independent of risk factors: Physical activity and cardiovascular health." NIH Consensus Development Conference Abstract, 77-83.

12. Blair, S. (1994). "Physical activity, fitness and coronary heart disease." In C. Bouchard, R.J. Shepard, & T. Stephens (Eds.), *Physical Activity, Fitness, and Health: International Proceedings and Consensus Statement.* (pp. 579-590). Champaign: Human Kinetics.

13. Paffenberger, R.S., Hyde, R.T., Wing, A.L., Lee, I.M., Jung, D. L., & Kampert, J.B. (1993). "The association of changes in physical activity level and other lifestyle characteristics with mortality among men." *New England Journal of Medicine* 328, 538-545.

14. Hagberg, J.M. (1995). "Physical activity, physical fitness, and blood pressure." NIH Consensus Development Conference Abstract, 69-71.

15. Orr, N., Dooly, C. (1999). "The Effects of Chronic Physical Activity on the Health and Fitness Profiles of Adults". *Medicine and Science in Sport and Exercise* 31(5)134.

16. Stefanick, M.L. (1995). "Physical activity and lipid metabolism." NIH Consensus Development Conference Abstract, 65-67.

17. Lakka, T.A., Venalainen, J.M., Rauramaa, R., Salonen, R., Tuomilehto, J., & Salonen, J.T. (1994). "Relation of leisure-time physical activity and cardiorespiratory fitness to the risk of acute myocardial infarction." *New England Journal of Medicine* 330, 1549-1554.

18. Bouchard, C., Shephard, R.J., & Stephens, T. (Eds.). (1994). *Physical Activity, Fitness, and Health.* Champaign: Human Kinetics.

19. Nieman, D.C. (2003). *Exercise Testing and Prescription a Health Related Approach.* (pp. 384-385). New York, NY: McGraw-Hill Higher Education.

20. Frohlich, E.D. (1994). "Hypertension." In T.A. Pearson, M.H. Criqui, R.K. Luepker, A. Oberman, & M. Winston (Eds.), *AHA Primer in Preventive Cardiology.* (pp. 131-142). Dallas: American Heart Association.

21. World Health Organization. (2000). "Obesity: preventing and managing the global epidemic." Report of a WHO consultation. *World Health Organ Tech Rep Ser* 894:1-253.

22. Berg, F.M. (1992). "Health risks of obesity: 1993 special report." *Obesity and Health.* Hettinger, ND.

23. Elmer, P.J. (1994). "Obesity in cardiovascular disease: Practical approaches for weight loss in clinical practice." In T.A. Pearson, M.H. Criqui, R.K. Luepker, A. Oberman, & M. Winston (Eds.), *AHA Primer in Preventive Cardiology.* (pp. 189-204). Dallas: American Heart Association.

24. Livengood, J.R., Casperton, C.J., & Koplan, J.P. (1993). "The health benefits of exercise." *New England Journal of Medicine* 328, 1852-58.

25. Orr, N., Dooly, C. (2001). "The Effects of Exercise Duration on Cardiovascular Disease Risk Factors: A Comparison of Two Groups", *Medicine and Science in Sport and Exercise* 33(5)4.

26. Orr, N., Dooly, C. (2000). "The Effects of a University Based Employee Health Promotion Program on Cardiovascular Risk Profiles" *Medicine and Science in Sport and Exercise* 32(5)126.

27. Cyr, N. (2002). "Exercise Benefits and Physiological Changes in Sedentary Adults," *American Journal of Health Promotion* 16(6)362.

28. Gotto, A.M. (1994). "Lipid and lipoprotein disorders." In T.A. Pearson, M.H. Criqui, R.K. Luepker, A. Oberman, & M. Winston (Eds.), *AHA Primer in Preventive Cardiology.* (pp. 107-129). Dallas: American Heart Association.

29. Bryant, S. (1990). "Exercise intervention for CHD. Cardiovascular Disease: Nutrition for prevention and treatment." *Journal of the American Dietetic Association* 90, 192-224.

30. U.S. Department of Health and Human Services. (1990). *Healthy People 2000 National Health Promotion and Disease Prevention Objectives.* (DHHS Publication No. PHS 91-50213). Washington, DC: Government Printing Office.

31. Becker, D.M. (1994). "Clinical approaches to cardiovascular risk factors: smoking." In T.A. Pearson, M.H. Criqui, R.K. Luepker, A. Oberman, & M. Winston (Eds.), *AHA Primer in Preventive Cardiology.* (pp. 143-145). Dallas: American Heart Association.

32. Hermanson, B., Omenn, G.S., Kronmal, R.A. & Gersh, B.J. (1988). "Beneficial six-year outcome of smoking cessation in older men and women with coronary artery disease. Results from the CASS Registry." *New England Journal of Medicine* 319, 1365-1369.

33. Paffenberger, R.S., & Hale, W.E. (1975). "Work activity and coronary heart mortality." *New England Journal of Medicine* 292, 545-550.

34. Blair, S.N., Kohl III, H.W., Paffenberger, R.S., Clark, G.G., Cooper, K.H., & Gibbons, L.W. (1989). "Physical fitness and all-cause mortality." *Journal of the American Medical Association* 262, 2395-2401.

35. McArdle, W.D., Katch, F.I., & Katch, V.L. (2001). *Exercise Physiology: Energy, Nutrition, and Human Performance.* (5th ed., pp. 922-934). Boston: Williams and Wilkins.

36. Fletcher, G.F., Blair, S., Blumenthal, J. (1992). "AHA statement on exercise: Benefits and recommendations for physical activity programs for all Americans." *Circulation* 86, 340-44.

37. Mercer-Meidinger, W. (1985). "Employer attitudes toward the cost of health: A William-Meidinger Survey." New York: William Mercer-Meidinger

38. Moy, C Moretz, S. (1988). "Wellness Programs: Keeping Workers Fit." *Occupational Hazards* 60, 59-62.

39. Chenoweth, D.H. (1991). *Planning Health Promotion at the Worksite.* (2nd ed., p. 12). Dublique, IA: Brown and Benchmark.

40. Chenoweth, D.H. (1998). *Worksite Health Promotion.* (pp. 5-11). New Bern, NC: Human Kinetics.

41. Katzman, M.S. & Smith, K.J. (1989). "Occupational health promotion programs: Evaluation efforts and measured cost savings." *Health Values* 13, 3-10.

42. Chapman, L.S. (1995). "Meta-Analysis of Studies on the Cost-Effectiveness of Worksite Health Promotion Programs." Paper presented at the annual meeting of the American Journal of Health Promotion, Orlando, FL.

43. Goetzel, R.Z., Juday, T.R., Ozminkowski, R. (1999). "What's The ROI?" *Association of Worksite Health Promotion Worksite Health.* Summer, 12-21.

44. Shi, L. (1992). "The impact of increasing intensity of health promotion intervention on risk reduction." *Evaluation and the Health Professionals* 15, 3-25.

45. Caspersen, C.J., Powell, K.E., & Christenson, G.M. (1987). "Physical activity and coronary heart disease." *The Physician and Sports Medicine* 15, 43-44.

46. Leon, A.S. (1995). "Contributions of regular moderate-intensity physical activity to reduced risk of coronary heart disease. Physical activity and cardiovascular health." NIH Consensus Development Abstract, 41-48.

47. Paffenberger, R.S., Hyde, R.T., Wing, A.L., Lee, I.M., Jung, D. L., & Kampert, J.B. (1993). "The association of changes in physical activity level and other lifestyle characteristics with mortality among men." *New England Journal of Medicine* 328, 538-545.

48. Romijn, J.A., Coyle, E.F., & Sidossis, L.S. et al. (1993). "Regulation of endogenous fat carbohydrate metabolism in relation to exercise intensity and duration." *American Journal of Physiology,* 265 (Endocranial. Metabolism 28), E380-391.

49. Orr, N. (1997). "Effects of a Health Promotion Program on Select Cardiovascular Risk Factors." *American Journal of Health Promotion* 11(6)445.

CHAPTER TWO

EPIDEMIOLOGY AND PATHOPHYSIOLOGY OF CARDIOVASCULAR DISEASE

This chapter reviews the epidemiology and pathophysiology of cardiovascular disease (CVD). Special attention is given to CVD prevalence and incidence data, and to the biological origin and physiological progression of atherosclerosis.

Despite a progressive decline in the death rate from coronary heart disease (CHD) since 1968, it remains the leading cause of death in the United States and is a major contributor to disability, lost productivity, and medical costs.[1] Since 1980, advanced medical treatment, better diagnostic procedures, improved pharmacology and changes in lifestyle have helped reduce the death rate for CVD by 35% for all CVD, and 40% for CHD. Still, cardiovascular diseases, primarily coronary heart disease and stroke, kill as many Americans as all other diseases combined, and are leading contributors to premature disability. Each minute roughly two Americans die of CVD (one every 33 seconds), and overall about 40% of Americans die of CVD. Coronary heart diseases due to atherosclerosis, principally myocardial infarction, angina pectoris, and their sequelae, account for more than half (53%) of all CVD deaths. Other forms of heart disease, including arrhythmias, heart failure, hypertension, cardiopathy, and pulmonary embolism account for about 26% of CVD deaths. Stroke, the third leading cause of death in the United States, accounts for 13% of all U.S. deaths, and while a cerebral vascular accident (CVA) may manifest as an atherothrombotic brain infarction, a cerebral embolism, an intra parenchymatous hemorrhage, a subarachnoid hemorrhage, or as a transient ischemic attack, the principal causative agent is related to atherosclerosis occurring in the arteries of the brain (Figure 2.1).[2-3]

The distribution of CVD rates by gender, sociocultural influences, race, and age provides valuable insight into its etiology. Heart disease rates are higher among men than women, but more women die from heart disease than men. In fact, heart disease is the leading cause of death in women. Research has demonstrated that women regard cancer as the number one cause of death, not heart disease. Additional research has also suggested that women may receive less aggressive medical treatment than men, even in those women who have had their first cardiac event, and that women are less likely than men to be evaluated for cardiovascular disease risk factors.

Heart disease death rates are higher among African Americans than among Caucasians, and heart disease rates increase with age. From the Framingham study, it has been established that CHD develops in men 60 years of age or younger at approximately twice the rate as in women.[2,4-5] Racial differences in the presentation of CHD have documented higher rates among African Americans as compared to Caucasians, in both males and females. African American men suffer an age-adjusted coronary heart disease death rate of 208 per 100,000 as compared to 185 per 100,000 in Caucasian men.[2] Due to variability among nations, epidemiological evidence suggests a strong genetic predisposition for the progression

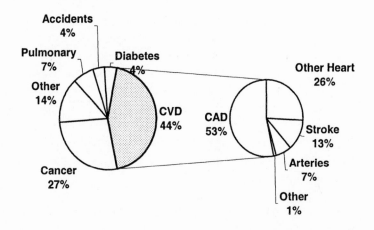

FIGURE 2.1 – The pie chart on the left shows the number one cause of premature death and disability is cardiovascular disease (CVD). As depicted in the pie chart on the right, coronary artery disease (CAD) is the primary contributor to CVD.

of CVD combined with powerful environmental and lifestyle influences. Migration studies have demonstrated that when people relocate from geographical regions where CVD rates are lower to regions where CVD rates are higher, the powerful influences of the adopted culture overpower the genetic influences, leading to higher CVD rates. This evidence further strengthens the relationship between the powerful influences of lifestyle choices and CVD rates.[6]

For both men and women, the incidence of CVD increases with age and is the leading cause of illness, disability, and death among those aged 65 and older.[4,7] In men, the highest incidence of clinical manifestations of CVD occurs between the ages of 40 and 60. In women, the highest incidence of CVD is between 60 and 70.[8]

PATHOPHYSIOLOGY OF CARDIOVASCULAR DISEASE

The underlying cause of 85% of all CVD, and the precursor to the clinical manifestation of CVD is atherosclerosis.[2] Atherosclerosis results from complex pathological processes that affect different arteries and certain sites within an artery more than others. Isolated in infants, the clinical symptoms of atherosclerosis usually manifest themselves in the fourth to fifth decade of life in men and approximately a decade later in women. Multiple physiological alterations influenced by genetics and lifestyle choices can act synergistically to accelerate or retard the progression of atherosclerosis [9] (Figure 2.2).

The primary physiological indicators that affect arterial structure, function, and consequentially, blood flow are evident from infancy to late adulthood. Composed of foam cells and termed fatty streaks, they line the intima of the vessel wall and have been identified in almost all population groups regardless of the prevalence of CVD. According to St. Clair, this may suggest that only some fatty streaks are precursors of more advanced atherosclerotic plaques or that risk factors and genetic factors may accelerate the progression of fatty streaks to plaques rather than promote their initial formation.[9]

Fatty streaks develop into fatty plaques and constitute the most recognizable lesions of atherosclerosis. Forming between the first and third decade of life, the fatty plaques are comprised mostly of lipids. An internal core of collagen, elastin and connective cells surrounds the plaque and gives it a fibrous cap.[10-11] The central core of the plaque contains mainly a lipid material with various plasma components including white blood cells, albumin, fibrin, fibrinogen, and cellular debris.[8] Considerable research utilizing animal models has established that certain components of the atherosclerotic lesion can be made to regress.[12] This process requires extensive lifestyle modification and intervention, and necessitates a serum cholesterol level of well below 200 mg/dl.[9] Most pathologists believe that lifestyle modifications can slow the progression of the atherosclerotic lesion.[12-13]

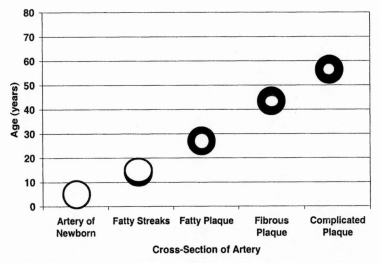

FIGURE 2.2 – The progression of atherosclerosis.

Complicated plaques become evident in the later part of the third decade of life and represent the "clinical horizon" of atherosclerosis.[9] The discriminating feature of the complicated plaque is evidence of rupture, mineralization, internal hemorrhage, calcification, necrosis, ulceration or thrombus formation over the plaque.[8-10,14] Calcification of longstanding lesions is common and can contribute to stiff, noncompliant vessels.[10,15]

As the lumen becomes less compliant, it loses its ability to dilate and constrict. The ability of the vessel to locally dilate and constrict is most likely regulated by either intrinsic neural control or by nutrient demand. These two theories have been explained by Guyton.[16] The first theory, called the vasodilator theory, proposes that a vasodilator substance is responsible for local regulation of blood flow. Possible agents include adenosine, carbon dioxide, lactic acid, adenosine phosphate compounds, histamine, potassium ions, and hydrogen ions. It is believed that adenosine may be the most important. The theory postulates that the substance is released from the tissue in response to oxygen deficiency and through a feedback mechanism diffuses back to the precapillary sphincter to cause dilation. The second theory postulates that local blood flow is regulated primarily by oxygen and other nutrient demands. This theory states that appropriate vasomotion (constriction and dilation) occurs locally in response to oxygen (and other nutrient) needs.

Humoral regulation is achieved through substances, such as hormones, that are released or secreted into the bloodstream to cause vasoconstriction or vasodilation. Norepinephrine is a powerful vasoconstrictor and epinephrine a less powerful vasoconstrictor that may even cause vasodilation under certain circumstances (usually myocardial vasodilation) in response to increased heart activity. Angiotensin is a potent vasoconstrictor that increases arterial resistance and, therefore, total peripheral resistance. Vasopressin (anti-diuretic hormone, or ADH) is a more powerful vasoconstrictor than angiotensin and is perhaps the most powerful constrictor in the body. The main function of vasopressin is to play a significant role in regulating body fluid volume. Vasodilators include bradykinin, serotonin, histamine, and prostaglandins. Other ions and chemical agents can also have vasoconstriction or vasodilation effects on local arterioles including calcium, potassium, magnesium, sodium, and anions acetate and citrate. An increase in hydrogen ions, and a decrease in pH can cause dilation, and a decrease in hydrogen ions can cause constriction.[16]

Regardless of the local or systemic mechanism, the net result of inadequate vasomotion is decreased blood flow and, therefore, decreased oxygen delivery. As a result, systemic and myocardial blood supply can be compromised. Also, since normal myocardial oxygen uptake extracts 70% - 80% of the oxygen supplied for use by myocardial tissue, myocardial oxygen uptake cannot increase significantly. As the amount of blood flow through the myocardium or peripheral vessel decreases, decreased oxygen supply to the tissues becomes evident.[10,15,17] As a result, the affected organ suffers from an ischemic condition.

Progressive and prolonged ischemia can result in necrosis of tissue. As central and peripheral hemodynamics continue to become compromised, clinical symptoms such as angina pectoris and peripheral ischemia become evident. Initially, individuals with atherosclerosis may be asymptomatic, but as the lesion develops and the vessel becomes occluded, clinical symptoms will arise. While symptoms usually correlate with lesions that occlude at least 60-75% of the vascular supply to an area, the development of collateral circulation may limit the level of ischemia, or decreased function.[10,14-15,18]

While the clinical pathology of atherosclerosis is relatively clear, the pathogenesis of atherosclerosis is less clear. Six plausible hypotheses are accepted in the literature, some with congruent characteristics, each with multiple etiologies. The complexity of each hypothesis reflects the number of variables that are considered. Assuming that atherosclerosis is a complex pathological process, environmental, genetic, and lifestyle characteristics must be accounted for, each with varying intensities. The two hypotheses that receive the most attention in the literature are the monoclinal hypothesis and the response to injury hypothesis, with the response to injury hypothesis receiving the most credibility.[8-9,14]

The response to injury hypothesis was first proposed by Virchow and later revised by Ross and Glomset.[9] The hypothesis postulates that as a result of microtrauma in the intima, a loss of endothelial cells ensues. Endothelial cells line the intima and are responsible for a number of functions and contribute to others including the regulation of the uptake of macromolecules. Damage to these cells may alter lipoprotein metabolism and/or retard specific lipoprotein transport mechanisms. The microtrauma may precipitate excessive serum lipoproteins or modifications in lipid structure that may exacerbate atherosclerosis. Causative contributors to the microtrauma can be of mechanical, chemical, hormonal, or immunologic stressors, and may include hydrocarbons from cigarette smoke, circulating cholesterol, and turbulence from blood flowing through hypertensive vessels.[8]

Platelet aggregation follows, and substances may be released (platelet derived growth factor) that may interact with plasma constituents and cause a proliferation of smooth muscle cells which form new connective tissue within the intima. Years of continuous blood flow, turbulence, and excessive serum lipoproteins can result in additional microtrauma and subsequent proliferation of smooth muscle cells that reinforce the injured site creating a complicated plaque.

Modifications to the theory have included studies that have shown that endothelial cell loss and platelet adhesion are not typically associated with the early phases of atherosclerosis, but appear later, usually after complicated plaques are present.[9] Other research has shown that macrophages, not smooth muscle cells, predominate in early lesions in humans as well as in animals.[19-20] St. Clair has redefined the nature of the injury as a more subtle form of endothelial cell dysfunction.[9] This is a result of data that has suggested that a variety of agents, from viruses to hyperlipidemias, have been associated with accelerated atherosclerosis, perhaps because of their common ability to modulate endothelial cell function.

The clinical manifestations of atherosclerosis can occur in the coronary arteries and/or in the peripheral vasculature. The vessels that appear to be most susceptible to atherosclerosis are the aorta, the coronary, carotid, and iliac arteries.[10] Coronary artery disease, the leading contributor to CVD, can manifest itself with four different clinical symptoms: (a) angina; (b) myocardial infarction; (c) sudden cardiac death; and, (d) congestive heart failure.[14,21] Systemically, the clinical consequences of atherosclerosis include a cerebral infarction, gangrene of the extremities, or an abdominal or aortic aneurism.[8] The rate of progression and clinical manifestations of atherosclerosis are not predictable or stable and are most likely affected by the vessel involved, the site of the lesion, and the age, genetic makeup, lifestyle, and physiologic status of the individual.[22]

REFERENCES

1.   American Heart Association. *2001 Heart and Stroke Statistical Update: Heart and Stroke Facts.* Dallas: American Heart Association, 2001.

2. Nieman, D.C. (2003). Exercise Testing and Prescription a Health Related Approach. (pp. 363-417). New York, NY: McGraw-Hill Higher Education.

3. Centers for Disease Control and Prevention. *The Promise of Prevention. Reducing the Health and Economic Burden of Chronic Disease.* Atlanta: Department of Health and Human Services, Centers for Disease Control and Prevention, February, 2003.

4. Thurber, K. (1990). "Risk factors for coronary heart disease." *Cardiovascular Disease: Nutrition for Prevention and Treatment.* American Dietetic Association, 1,33.

5. Luepker, R.V. (1994). "Epidemiology of atherosclerotic diseases in population groups." In T.A. Pearson, M.H. Criqui, R.K. Luepker, A. Oberman, & M. Winston (Eds.), *AHA Primer in Preventive Cardiology.* (pp. 1-10). Dallas: American Heart Association.

6. Kagan, A., Harris, B.R., Winkelstein, W., Johnson, K.G., Kato, H., Syme, S.L., Rhoads, G.G., Gay, M.L., Nichaman, M.Z., Hamilton, H.B., & Tillotson, J. (1974). "Epidemiologic studies of coronary heart disease and stroke in Japanese men living in Japan, Hawaii, and California: Demographic, physical, dietary, and biochemical characteristics." *Journal of Chronic Diseases* 27, 345-364.

7. Middlemark, M.B., Pasty, B.M., & Rautaharju, P.M., et al. (1993). "Prevalence of cardiovascular disease among older adults." *American Journal of Epidemiology* 137, 311-317.

8. Brannon, F.J., Foley, M.W., Starr, J.A., & Black, M.G. (1993). *Cardiopulmonary Rehabilitation: Basic Theory and Practice.* (2nd ed., pp. 84-85). Philadelphia: F. A. Davis.

9. St. Clair, R.W. (1983). "Atherosclerosis regression in animal models: Current concepts of cellular and biochemical mechanisms." *Progressive Cardiovascular Disease* 26, 109-132.

10. Bullock, B.L., & Rosenthal, P.P. (1992). *Pathophysiology: Adaptations and Alterations in Function* (3rd ed., pp. 538-540). Philadelphia: J.B. Lippincott.

11. Cowan, M. (1986). "Atherosclerosis." In M.L. Patrick, et al. (Eds.), *Medical Surgical Nursing: Pathophysiological Concepts.* Philadelphia: J.B. Lippincott.

12. St. Clair, R.W. (1983). "Atherosclerosis regression in animal models: Current concepts of cellular and biochemical mechanisms." *Progressive Cardiovascular Disease* 26, 109-132.

13. Ross, R., & Glosmet, J.A. (1976). "The pathogenesis of atherosclerosis, Part I." *New England Journal of Medicine, 259,* 369.

14. McCance, K.L., & Huether, S.E. (1994). *Pathophysiology.* (2nd ed., p. 1018). St. Louis: Mosby.

15. Price, S.A., & Wilson, L.M. (1992). *Pathophysiology: Clinical concepts of disease process.* (4th ed., pp. 81-83). St. Louis: Mosby.

16. Guyton, A.C. (1991). *Textbook of Medical Physiology* (8th ed., pp. 761-763). Philadelphia: W.B. Saunders.

17. McArdle, W.D., Katch, F.I., & Katch, V.L. (2001). *Exercise Physiology: Energy, Nutrition, and Human Performance.* (5th ed., pp. 320-321). Boston: Williams and Wilkins.

18. Fowler, N.O. (Ed.). (1980). *Cardiac Diagnosis and Treatment.* Hagerstown, MD: Harper and Row.

19. Stary, H.C. (1990). "The sequence of cell and matrix changes in atherosclerosis lesions of coronary arteries in the forty years of life." *European Heart Journal* 11(suppl. E), 3-19.

20. Masuda, J., & Ross, R. (1990). "Atherogenesis during low level hypercholesterolemia in the nonhuman primate: I. fatty streak formation." *Arteriosclerosis and Thrombosis* 10, 164-177.

21. Vinsant, M.O., & Spence, M.I. (1988). *Common Sense Approach to Coronary Care: A Program.* (5th ed.). St. Louis: Mosby.

22. Haak, S.W., Richardson, S.J., Davey, S.S., & Parker-Cohen, P.D. (1994). "Alterations in cardiovascular function." *Pathophysiology.* (pp. 1000-1084). St. Louis: Mosby.

CHAPTER THREE

PHYSIOLOGICAL MECHANISMS AND CAUSATIVE FACTORS OF CARDIOVASCULAR DISEASE

This chapter explains the relationship between the biological foundation and physiological progression of CVD risk factors to the clinical manifestation of CVD. Physiological pathways and biological mechanisms are explored.

The genetic and lifestyle influences that can accelerate the progression of atherosclerosis are collectively termed risk factors, because past and present research has demonstrated their association with higher rates of CVD. Risk factors are derived from a mathematical analysis of the relative risk of a person developing CVD with a specific risk factor as compared to the risk of a second person absent of that particular risk factor. The relative risk of major risk factors for CVD is about 2.0. This means that a person with one CVD risk factor has the chance of developing CVD at twice the rate of a second person absent that particular risk factor.

Major CVD risk factors include:

- hypercholesterolemia
- diabetes
- hypertension
- cigarette smoking
- obesity
- inactivity

Classified as either unmodifiable (genetics [i.e. heredity, family history], gender, and age) or modifiable risk factors (hypercholesterolemia, diabetes, hypertension, cigarette smoking, obesity, and inactivity), they have been catalogued as markers and are used to determine cardiovascular disease risk profiles. The physiological mechanisms and causative factors that tie the risk factors to CVD encompass a multitude of physiological alterations in biochemical, hormonal, and physiological regulatory processes. Risk factors are not created equally: each has its own etiology and pathology, and each can be influenced by a unique combination of lifestyle, genetics, and environmental factors. Therefore, individual variability is common, plausible, and natural. The combination of risk factors may have a potentiating effect on CHD risk (Figure 3.1).

Genetics, perhaps the strongest unmodifiable biological characteristic, plays an important role in the predisposition for certain conditions including lipid abnormalities, hypertension, obesity, and CVD. First degree relatives of early CHD patients are at much higher risk for developing CHD than the general population.[1-2] Williams determined that a strong family predisposition to early coronary heart disease occurs in approximately 5% of the general population of families; however, the coronary-prone families accounted for more than 50% of the cases of coronary disease occurring before the age of 55.[2] According to Oberman, and Nieman, a strong family history of premature CAD before the age of 55 in first degree relatives corresponds to between two and five times the risk of those without this history.[3-4] Bullock

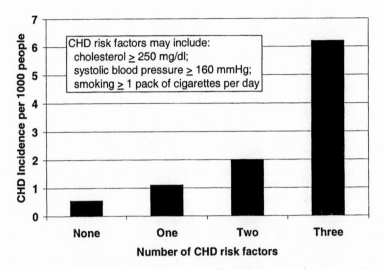

FIGURE 3.1 – The relationship between the number of risk factors and the incidence of CHD. *Source:* McArdle, W D, Katch, FI, & Katch, V L. *Exercise Physiology: Energy, Nutrition and Human Performance (5th ed.).* p. 904. Boston: Lippincott, Williams and Wilkins, 2001.

determined that the genetic predisposition for the development of CHD is increased further when a strong family history is combined with other risk factors.[1] Hunt further delineated the influence of genetics and computed relative risk ratios when the incidence of CAD is evident in first degree relative(s) and clinically manifests at an earlier age.[5] As depicted in Figure 3.2, the author derived a relative risk of 12.7 for men aged 20-39, and 12.9 for women aged 40-49 when a positive family history is evident in two first degree relatives prior to age 55. The relative risk shrinks to 3.9 (men) and 2.5 (women) when a positive family history is evident in one first degree relative prior to age 55.

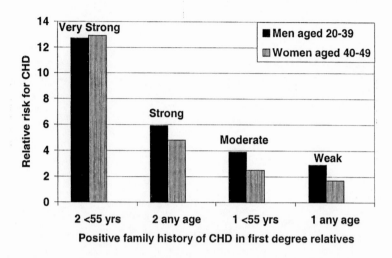

FIGURE 3.2 – The relationship between a positive family history of CHD in first degree relatives and the relative risk for CHD. *Source:* Hunt, SC, Williams, RR, & Barlow, BK. A comparison of positive family history definitions for defining risk of future disease. *Journal of Chronic Diseases*, 1986;69:809-821.

Hyperlipidemia, especially hypercholesterolemia, is associated with premature CVD. The strong relationship to premature CVD is suggestive of congenital abnormalities of lipid-metabolizing enzymes, overproduction of lipids and/or abnormal cellular receptors and is related to, and often a consequence of, high saturated fat intake.[6] An elevated level of HDL cholesterol is believed to serve as a cardioprotective agent and is inversely related to CHD risk. The inverse relationship is related to the role of HDL cholesterol as HDL cholesterol facilitates reverse cholesterol transport by promoting the removal of cholesterol from the peripheral tissues to the liver for biosynthesis.[7]

Numerous factors affect plasma lipoprotein levels including age, gender, diet, weight, diabetes, smoking, antihypertensive agents, exogenous hormones, and exercise.[8] The ratio of total cholesterol (TC) to high density lipoproteins (HDL) has been used as a predictor for CHD. Risk increases when the ratio exceeds 4.5 for men and 4.0 for women with an optimal ratio for low CVD risk established when the ratio of total cholesterol to high density lipoproteins (TC:HDL) is below 3.5.[9] The ratio of TC to HDL cholesterol should not be used as a primary indicator, but should be used in conjunction with other plasma lipid values, especially since LDL cholesterol has been classified as the atherogenic lipoprotein. While hyperlipidemia is a risk factor for premature CHD, dyslipidemia has also been closely associated with diabetes.

Research has demonstrated that type 2 diabetics (also referred to as non-insulin dependent diabetics or by the acronym NIDDM) are at an increased risk of premature CHD.[7-8] The relative risk of CHD complications in diabetics is similar to the relative risk of other traditionally known risk factors, such as hypertension, smoking, and hypercholesterolemia. Risk factors for both type 2 diabetes and CHD include age, inactivity, obesity, hypertension, smoking, dyslipidemia, and a central pattern of fat distribution.[10] As depicted in Table 3.1, many of the risk factors for Type 2 diabetes can be influenced by a healthy lifestyle.

TABLE 3.1 – Risk factors for type 2 diabetes

1. Inactivity
2. Body weight greater than 20% of recommended
3. Blood pressure $\geq$ 140/90 mmHg
4. HDL cholesterol $\leq$ 35 mg/dl and/or $\geq$ 250 triglyceride level
5. Diabetes in first degree relative
6. Impaired fasting blood glucose
7. High risk ethnic group
8. Gestational diabetes

Type 2 diabetes is a consequence of decreased insulin sensitivity, or insulin resistance, in peripheral tissues. A decrease in insulin sensitivity, or insulin resistance, is often due to a genetic predisposition exacerbated by obesity, poor dietary choices, and an overall poor level of physical fitness.[7] Cultural and ethnic prevalence differences provide insight into its etiology. American Indians and Alaska Natives are 2.8 times more likely to have diabetes than non-Hispanic whites, and African Americans are two times more likely than whites to die of diabetes.[4]

In 1994, more than 5% of adults had diabetes and 4.6% had some form of glucose intolerance, which means that almost a decade ago, about 10% of the population was diagnosed with some form of disturbed glucose tolerance.[10] Today, 6.5% of the population has type 2 diabetes, and another 8% have some type of impaired fasting glucose, a total of almost 15% of the population.

Type 2 diabetes accounts for 90% of all diabetics, and traditionally has occurred more frequently in adults.[7,10] In fact, one in five adults over the age of 65 has diabetes. The sixth leading cause of death in 1999, the direct and indirect medical costs of diabetes total almost $100 billion per year.[11] In 1997, the average annual health care cost to a person with diabetes was $10,000.00, as compared to $2,700.00 for a person without diabetes. From 1990 to 2000, the prevalence rates of type 2 diabetes increased from 4.9% to 6.5%, for a percentage increase of 33%. An estimated 15 million Americans have type 2 diabetes, and each year an additional 800,000 new cases of diabetes are diagnosed.[4] Another 20 million Americans have impaired fasting glucose, and 16 million U.S. adults aged 40-74 are classified as pre-diabetic. Associated with two modifiable risk factors, obesity and physical inactivity, the fastest growing segment of our population to be diagnosed with type 2 diabetes falls within the 30-39 age group. Because of its relationship to lifestyle choices and daily behaviors, and its dramatic increase in younger adults, public health officials have proclaimed type 2 diabetes as the fastest growing public health concern. As depicted in Figure 3.3, in the healthy reaction, insulin, a carrier hormone secreted by the pancreas in response to elevated blood glucose, transports glucose from the blood stream (capillary) to the peripheral tissue (muscle tissue), via the peripheral receptor. The glucose can now be catabolized, via aerobic or anaerobic pathways, to produce energy in the form of adenosine triphosphate (ATP). In the second illustration, referred to as pre-diabetic, the cellular receptor is becoming resistant to insulin. Therefore, insulin is less effective in transporting glucose from the bloodstream to the peripheral tissue, and the insulin remains elevated in the bloodstream. As the debilitating process continues, the receptor becomes down regulated, and insulin loses its effectiveness at transporting glucose into the peripheral tissue.

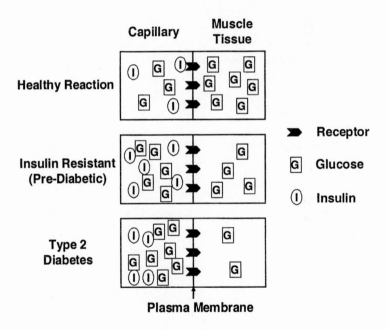

FIGURE 3.3 – The progression from a healthy glucose-insulin interaction (normal glucose uptake into peripheral tissue) to an insulin resistant (pre-diabetic) state, to type 2 diabetes (down-regulation of the peripheral receptors).

The clinical diagnosis of type 2 diabetes has traditionally occurred in adulthood, however, the relatively new increased incidence among young adults has shifted the diagnosis criteria away from age, and now focuses on symptoms and risk factor analysis. Criteria for the clinical diagnosis of diabetes mellitus in non-pregnant adults should be restricted to those who have one of the following:

(a) a fasting plasma glucose equal to or greater than 126 mg/dl (after no caloric intake after 8 hours);

(b) a casual fasting plasma glucose level (taken anytime of the day, without regard to time of last meal) that is equal to or greater than of 200 mg/dl, with the classic diabetes symptoms of increased urination, increased thirst, and unexplained weight loss;

(c) an oral glucose tolerance test (OGTT) value that is equal or greater than 200 mg/dl in the 2-hour sample.

The fasting plasma glucose test is the preferred and recommended test. A plasma glucose level of 60-109 mg/dl is normal. As illustrated in Table 3.2, stratification values for elevated risk are as follows: $\leq$109 mg/dl is normal fasting glucose; 110-125 mg/dl is categorized as impaired fasting glucose; and $\geq$ 126 mg/dl is clinically diagnosed as diabetes when confirmed on a separate day.

Unfortunately, excessive premature cardiovascular disease and related microvascular complications (retinopathy, neuropathy, nephropathy) are the usual consequences of diabetes.[12] Management of blood pressure is critical to the diabetic as chronic hypertension can exacerbate microvascular complications including retinopathy, neuropathy, and nephropathy.[10]

Hypertension, an elevation of arterial blood pressure, is regarded as a major risk factor for CVD. The National Institutes of Health has categorized hypertension according to severity of risk (Table 3.3). "Optimal" blood pressure is $\leq$120/80 mmHg. "Normal" blood pressure should be less than 130/85 mmHg, "high normal" is

TABLE 3.2 – Risk stratification for type 2 diabetes based upon blood glucose values

Classification	Blood Glucose (mg/dl)
Normal	< 109
Impaired	110-125
Diabetes	>126

TABLE 3.3 – Risk stratification for hypertension as based upon blood pressure values

Classification	Blood Pressure (mmHg)
Optimal	≤ 120/80
Pre-Hypertension	(120-140)/(80-90)
Normal	130/85
High Normal	(130-139)/(85-89)
Hypertension	140/90
Stage 1 Hypertension	(140-159)/(90-99)
Stage 2 Hypertension (moderate)	(160-179)/(100-109)
Stage 3 Hypertension (severe)	(180-209)/(110-119)
Stage 4 Hypertension (very severe)	> 210/120

defined as a reading of 130-139/85-89 mmHg, and "hypertension" is categorized above 140/90 mmHg. Due to the severity of hypertension and its prevalence rates, new language has been instituted to describe any blood pressure value that falls between 120/80 mmHg, and 140/90 mmHg. The new descriptor, which affects 45 million Americans, is pre-hypertension, and it denotes the significance of an increased blood pressure value and its relationship to hypertension. Stage 1 hypertension is defined as a blood pressure reading above 140/90 mmHg, and between 140-159/90-99 mmHg. Stage 2, or moderate hypertension is a blood pressure reading that falls between 160-179/100-109 mmHg. Stage 3, or severe hypertension, is 180-209/110-119 mmHg, and very severe hypertension, or stage 4, is above 210/120 mmHg. It is important to note, however, that regardless of which reference points are utilized, the higher the systolic and diastolic blood pressure, the higher cardiovascular morbidity, and mortality rates.

The prevalence of hypertension increases with age and is higher for less educated people.[13] In 2000, 28% of adults, (50 million people) in the U.S. were hypertensive (age-adjusted to the year 2000 standard population), and another 30 million adults have high normal blood pressure.[4] Hypertension is greater in younger and middle-aged men as compared to women (age range 20-54), but greater in older women as compared to men (age >55). 57.3% of men and 60.8% of women aged 65-74 are hypertensive, and 64.2% of men, and 77.3% of women are hypertensive after age 75.[4] Hypertension is higher among African Americans and Hispanic Americans as compared to Caucasians.[13] During the past several decades, the incidence of hypertension has decreased as both systolic and diastolic blood pressure values have declined in all age, sex, and race subgroups except African American men over the age of 50.

Predisposing factors include heredity and lifestyle, with hyperlipidemia and subsequent obesity being major risk factors.[1,14] Other contributors include: alcohol intake, inactivity, sodium intake, and smoking.[4] Hypertension has been known to contribute to a multitude of pathological conditions including cerebrovascular events, CAD, congestive heart failure, and renal disease. While the etiology of hypertension is unclear and unknown in up to 95% of all hypertensive individuals, the baseline trait is an increase in total peripheral resistance (TPR) at rest. TPR is the sum of all resistances offered by the vascular beds of the body. While these may vary with different organs, systemic peripheral resistance has the greatest effect on the mean arterial blood pressure.[1] Blood pressure is a product of vessel diameter (the precapillary sphincter diameter) and cardiac output (the product of heart rate and stroke volume).

Several theories have been offered to explain essential hypertension including:

   (a) chronic changes in the arteriolar bed causing increased resistance;

(b) abnormally increased tone of the sympathetic nervous system (SNS) from the vasomotor centers causing increased peripheral vascular resistance (PVR);

(c) increased blood volume resulting from renal or hormonal dysfunction; and,

(d) a genetic increase in arteriolar thickening causing abnormal PVR. Most researchers believe the etiology is complex and multifactorial.[1,14]

Renal sodium metabolism, regulated by the kidneys and influenced by hormones (renin, angiotensin, aldosterone, atrial natriuretic factor, prostaglandins, and insulin), is believed to play a dominant role in maintaining the increased blood pressure in essential hypertension because the appropriate regulation of sodium metabolism is essential to maintaining plasma volume and cardiac output.[15] There is also evidence to suggest that a connection exists between the SNS and hypertension due to circulating plasma norepinephrine levels, which may increase peripheral vascular resistance and contractility.[16] The SNS also influences the renin-angiotensin-aldosterone (RAA) system, which causes arteriolar constriction through the release of angiotensin II and increased blood volume through the liberation of aldosterone.[1]

The long term effects of hypertension alter the structure of the heart and consequentially affect cardiovascular dynamics. Chronic hypertension creates increased afterload which brings about increased pressure in the ventricle. In response to the increased pressure, additional muscle mass develops, creating concentric ventricular hypertrophy or enlargement from the epicardium to the endocardium. While the chamber size does not increase in size, the thicker myocardium becomes heavier. The thicker and heavier heart experiences increased myocardial oxygen requirements, and suffers from decreased compliance. Coronary atherosclerosis is exacerbated by the increased oxygen demand and increased blood flow, which precipitates premature angina, ischemia, and infarction.[1]

Prolonged systemic hypertension causes excessive pressure on small vessel arterioles, which leads to organ dysfunction. The main organ casualties of chronic essential hypertension include the heart, eyes, brain, and kidneys.[14] The clinical manifestations in the heart include myocardial infarction, congestive heart failure, myocardial hypertrophy, and dysrhythmia. The eyes suffer from blurred or impaired vision and/or encephalopathy and the brain suffers from cerebral vascular events (CVA) and also encephalopathy. Subsequent kidney damage including renal insufficiency and renal failure are also consequences of chronic systemic hypertension.[1,14]

Smoking and tobacco use are lifestyle related learned behaviors that are strong and independent risk factors for all types of CVD (CHD, stroke, and peripheral artery disease). Smoking and tobacco use are the single most preventable cause of premature death in the U.S. today, and direct medical costs attributed to smoking total more than $75 billion per year.[11] Approximately 24% of U.S. adults currently smoke or use tobacco, and a total of almost 20% of all deaths are the result of cigarette smoking.[4] The prevalence of smoking has declined since the 1960's, but has leveled off somewhat during the 1990's. The optimistic goal in Healthy People 2010 is to reduce the percentage of smokers to 12% of the population. More men than women smoke, and among subgroups American Indians, and Alaska Natives smoke at a prevalence rate of 40%. White, non-Hispanic and black non-Hispanics smoke at a similar reported rate of about 24%, and Hispanics smoke at a rate of 19.1%. Asian and Pacific Islanders smoke the least, a rate of 13.7%. People falling in the lower socioeconomic subgroups (SES) smoke more than those in higher SES subgroups. Research studies have indicated that within the congregate of people who have ever smoked on a daily basis, 82% tried their first cigarette prior to age 18.[17]

Research has documented that smokers develop peripheral atherosclerosis at a rate of two to five times more often than those who have never smoked.[18] A clear correlation exists between smoking and increased CHD risk, with a dose-response relationship between number of cigarettes smoked and CHD risk.[7,19] Cigarette smoking has consistently been associated with CHD, stroke, sudden death, and peripheral vascular disease and, consequentially, has resulted in higher morbidity and mortality rates.[19-20] Studies indicate that 87% of all lung cancers can be directly attributed to smoking.[21]

Whereas Haak[6] and Carleton[20] postulate that the effect of nicotine on catecholamine (epinephrine and norepinephrine) release by the autonomic nervous system appears to be the mechanism responsible, Becker believes that the relationship between smoking and cardiovascular disease results from "multiple mechanisms acting synergistically to cause endothelial injury, an abnormal intravascular environment, and abnormalities in both the electrical conducting system and the function of ventricular myocardium."[19]

Specifically, nicotine stimulates the release of epinephrine and norepinephrine causing increased heart rate and peripheral vascular constriction resulting in increased blood pressure.[6] Elevated blood nicotine levels have been associated with arterial endothelial injury.[19] Cigarette gas and vapor components including carbon monoxide and nicotine have been linked to clotting and platelet factors that predispose to thrombus formation, vascular smooth muscle proliferation, and the subsequent development of complex vascular lesions.[6,19] Carbon monoxide has also been associated with lowered oxygen content in arterial blood.[6] Platelet adhesiveness and aggregation, acute and chronic coronary vasoconstriction along with increased fibrinogen levels and decreased plasminogen have been associated with smoking.[1,19]

Cigarette smoking increases heart rate and blood pressure, therefore, increasing myocardial oxygen demands and may also lower the threshold for ventricular arrhythmias.[6,19] Research has documented that smokers have lower serum levels of HDL cholesterol and some agents in cigarette smoke contain substances that have deleterious effects on the ventricular myocardium.[1,7,19]

Another risk factor for CVD is being overweight or obese. The prevalence of obesity increases with age and is one of the most prevalent health problems in the United States. The World Health Organization, and the National Heart, Lung, and Blood Institute have classified obesity as an epidemic. The rates of obesity have increased across all subgroups of the American population. At 39%, the highest prevalence rates of obesity are found in African American females. 36% of Mexican-American females are obese, as well as 24% of white females, and Mexican American males. Prevalence rates among both white males and black males are 21%.[4]

Since 1960, the prevalence of obesity has nearly doubled from 13.3% in 1960 to 26% in 1999. The corresponding percentage of people who are either obese or overweight has dramatically increased from 1960-1999, with the percentage increasing from 44.8% to 61%. This has resulted in the percentage of the population who resides at a "healthy weight" to shrink from 51.2% in 1960 to 36% in 1999.[4]

Comparing the U.S. to other nations reveals alarming statistics. Citizens of the U.S. lead most of the world in the prevalence rates of obesity. Closely behind the U.S. are Mexico, The United Kingdom, and Russia. The lowest rates are found in Japan, China and Italy.[4]

As demonstrated in Figure 3.4, the rates of obesity have dramatically increased among children and young adults since the early 1960's. During that time, 4.2% of children aged 6-11 were obese, in 1999 the rate tripled to 13%. Young adults aged 12-19 demonstrated consistent three fold increases with 4.6% obese in the early 1960's, compared to 14% in 1999.[4] The consequence of this trend is the evident dramatic increases in the incidence of type 2 diabetes in our society, particularly within younger age groups.

Quantified by various measurements and calculations, obesity has been functionally defined by Thomas and adopted by the American Dietetic Association as a condition in which excess fat may put a person at health risk. [22] In the general population (excluding specific athletic groups), overweight has been defined as a BMI of between 25-29.9, and obesity has been defined as a BMI of greater then 30. Clinically, it increases the risk of developing hypertension, type 2 diabetes, and is an independent risk factor for CAD and stroke and is associated with hyperlipidemia.[4,23] Obesity has been linked to a variety of chronic diseases such as arthritis, certain types of cancer and gall bladder disease, and its consequences affect metabolic, orthopedic and cardiovascular functions.

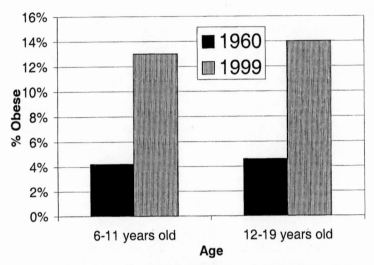

FIGURE 3.4 – The prevalence of obesity in youth, 1960-1999. *Source:* Nieman, David, C. *Exercise Testing and Prescription: A Health Related Approach.* p. 509. New York: McGraw-Hill, 2003

Excessive weight necessitates additional vasculature and blood supply that increases the metabolic requirements of the organism and consequentially increases myocardial work and total work load. As obesity progresses, myocardial hypertrophy occurs. Growing evidence is suggestive of a genetic component or predisposition to obesity.[1,7] Contributing factors to the increased prevalence of obesity include:

- increased portion size combined with a early childhood lesson to "finish everything on your plate"

- the abundant availability of appealing, and inexpensive food, and the multitude of food choices
- an advanced technological and automated society which makes movement less necessary
- decreases in opportunities to be active, including fewer sidewalks, and fewer playgrounds
- a decreased emphasis on the importance of daily physical activity

Other contributors include social, environmental, and perhaps racial influences, as well as hormonal imbalances, emotional trauma, and homeostatic imbalances.[7]

REFERENCES

1. Bullock, B.L., & Rosenthal, P.P. (1992). *Pathophysiology: Adaptations and Alterations in Function.* (3rd ed., pp. 148-149). Philadelphia: J.B. Lippincott.

2. Williams, R.R. (1984). "Understanding genetic and environmental risk factors in susceptible persons." *Western Journal of Medicine* 141, 799-806.

3. Oberman, A. (1989). "Epidemiology and prevention of cardiovascular disease." In W. N. Kelley (Ed.), *Textbook of Internal Medicine.* Philadelphia: J. B. Lippincott.

4. Nieman, D.C. (2003). *Exercise Testing and Prescription, a Health Related Approach.* (pp. 363-417, 477-546). New York, NY: McGraw-Hill Higher Education.

5. Hunt, S.C., Williams, R.R., & Barlow, B.K. (1986). "A comparison of positive family history definitions for defining risk of future disease." *Journal of Chronic Diseases* 69, 809-821.

6.   Haak, S.W., Richardson, S.J., Davey, S.S., & Parker-Cohen, P.D. (1994). "Alterations in cardiovascular function." *Pathophysiology*. (pp. 1000-1084). St. Louis: Mosby.

7.   McArdle, W.D., Katch, F.I., & Katch, V.L. (2001). *Exercise Physiology: Energy, Nutrition, and Human Performance*. (5th ed., pp. 26, 430-434). Boston: Williams and Wilkins.

8.   Kris-Etherton, P.M. (1990). *Cardiovascular Disease: Nutrition for Prevention and Treatment*. (p. 61). Chicago: The American Dietetic Association.

9.   Thurber, K. (1990). "Risk factors for coronary heart disease. Cardiovascular disease: Nutrition for prevention and treatment." American Dietetic Association, 1, 33.

10. Orchard, T.J., (1994). "Diabetes." In T.A. Pearson, M.H. Criqui, R.K. Luepker, A. Oberman, and M. Winston (Eds.), *AHA Primer in Preventive Cardiology*. (pp. 159-171). Dallas: American Heart Association.

11. Centers for Disease Control and Prevention. *The Promise of Prevention. Reducing the Health and Economic Burden of Chronic Disease*. Atlanta: Department of Health and Human Services, Centers for Disease Control and Prevention, February, 2003.

12. Donahue, R.P., & Orchard, T.J. (1992). "Diabetes mellitus and macrovascular complications. An epidemiological perspective." *Diabetes Care* 15, 1141-55.

13. Frohlich, E.D. (1994). "Hypertension." In T.A. Pearson, M.H. Criqui, R.K. Luepker, A. Oberman, & M. Winston (Eds.), *AHA Primer in Preventive Cardiology*. (pp. 131-142). Dallas: American Heart Association.

14. McCance, K.L., & Huether, S.E. (1994). *Pathophysiology*. (2nd ed., p. 1019). St. Louis: Mosby.

15. Hall, J.E., Mizelle, L., Hildebrandt, D.A., & Brands, M.W. (1990). "Abnormal pressure natriuresis: A cause or consequence of hypertension?" *Hypertension* 15, 547-559.

16. Molineux, D., & Steptoe, A. (1988). "Exaggerated blood pressure responses to submaximal exercise in normotensive adolescents with a family history of hypertension." *Journal of Hypertension* 6, 261-265.

17. U. S. Department of Health and Human Services. *Healthy People 2010.* [www.health.gov/healthypeople/]. Washington DC: January, 2002.

18. Criqui, M.H., Browner, D., Fvorek, A. Klauber, M.R., Coughlin, S.S., Barrett-Connor, E., & Gabriel, S. (1989). "Peripheral arterial disease in large vessels is epidemiologically distinct from small vessel disease: An analysis of risk factors." *American Journal of Epidemiology* 129, 1110-1119.

19. Becker, D.M. (1994). "Clinical approaches to cardiovascular risk factors: smoking." In T.A. Pearson, M.H. Criqui, R.K. Luepker, A. Oberman, & M. Winston (Eds.), *AHA Primer in Preventive Cardiology.* (pp. 143-145). Dallas: American Heart Association.

20. Carleton, P.F., & Boldt, M.A. (1992). "Coronary atherosclerotic disease." *Pathophysiology: Clinical Concepts of Disease Process.* (4th ed.). St. Louis: Mosby.

21. American Cancer Society. *Cancer Facts & Figures, 2001.* Atlanta: American Cancer Society, 2001.

22. Food and Nutrition Board, Institute of Medicine. P.R Thomas, Ed. (1995). *Weighing the Options: Criteria for Evaluating Weight Management Programs.* Committee to Develop Criteria for Evaluating the Outcome of Approaches to Prevent and Treat Obesity. Washington DC: National Academy Press.

23. Berg, F.M. (1992). "Health risks of obesity: 1993 special report." *Obesity and Health.* Hettinger, ND.

CHAPTER FOUR

PHYSIOLOGICAL MECHANISMS AND EXERCISE INTERVENTION

This chapter reviews the mechanisms whereby exercise, and physical activity affect the risk factors associated with CVD, thereby strengthening the body, and consequentially reducing CVD risk.

$\mathbf{W}$hile physical inactivity has been associated with increased all-cause mortality rates and higher clinical manifestations of CVD, regular physical activity has been linked with a decreased risk of CHD.[1-5] Regular physical activity improves CVD risk factors and other health-related factors, including blood lipid profiles, resting blood pressure in borderline hypertensives, body composition, cardiovascular fitness, glucose tolerance and insulin sensitivity, bone density, immune function, and psychological function.[5-6] The relative risk of CHD associated with physical inactivity ranges from 1.5 to 2.4 with a median of about 1.9.[4] This relative risk is comparable to the relative risk of hypercholesterolemia, hypertension, and smoking.[4,7]

The physiological mechanisms whereby physical activity reduces the relative risk for CHD have been extensively analyzed. In the 1980s, epidemiological studies suggested that regular activity may have directly affected the myocardium by retarding the atherosclerotic process, modifying the structure of the coronary arteries, reducing vasospasm, enhancing myocardial electrical stability, or increasing fibrinolysis.[4] Kemmer found that exercise improved glucose tolerance and insulin sensitivity and Seals determined that exercise assisted in weight control, and reduced blood pressure.[8-9] More recently, Haskell compiled a list of the biological mechanisms whereby exercise may contribute to the primary or secondary prevention of CHD.[3] The inclusive list details myocardial alterations that lead to either increased myocardial oxygen supply or decreased demand. The author states that all preventive and therapeutic measures for reducing clinical manifestations of CHD work through these mechanisms.

Specifically, participation in exercise programs may induce chronic adaptations that will occur within the cardiorespiratory (central) and peripheral systems. These adaptations will not only contribute to the primary and secondary prevention of CHD, but may also lead to an increase in performance.

At the present time, the best indicator of cardiorespiratory endurance is an assessment of maximal oxygen uptake (VO_2 max.). VO_2 max. is the product of stroke volume (SV), heart rate (HR), and a-vO_2 difference or cardiac output and a-vO_2 difference, referred to as the Fick equation.[10-11]

Evidence of increased cardiovascular efficiency is assessed through a higher VO_2 max. value. Wilmore found an average increase in VO_2 max. of 15-20% in sedentary persons following participation in an exercise program consisting of three times per week for 30 minutes at 75% of capacity.[10] This corresponds to an increase from 35 ml/kg/min to 42 ml/kg/min. Other researchers suggest an increase in VO_2 max. of between 5 and 30%.[12-14] Cardiorespiratory changes that lead to the increase in VO_2 max. include an increase in cardiac output due primarily through increased stroke volume.[10-11] Three factors enable stroke volume to increase: (a) increased venous return; (b) increased end-diastolic volume; and (c) increased contractility or greater systolic emptying.[10-11] Booth has subdivided the adaptations into those that alter stroke volume, and those that alter ejection fraction through changes in contractility (inotropic adaptations).[15] At lower workloads in an untrained person, the Frank Starling mechanism is the most important factor for maintaining cardiac output. At near maximal workloads (where end-diastolic volume cannot increase further), an increase in ejection fraction is necessary for an increase in cardiac output.

Changes in left ventricular size and chronotropic adaptations have been documented in response to endurance training.[15] The left ventricle undergoes internal changes as well as changes in size leading to eccentric hypertrophy.[16] Increases in left ventricular muscle mass, left ventricular end-diastolic diameter, and left ventricular septal and posterior wall thickness have been documented.[10-11] While the mechanism may not be completely clear, a decrease in exercising and resting heart rate (exercise induced bradycardia) due to increased parasympathetic activity in the heart and a corresponding decrease in sympathetic activity has been documented.[10-11,15] According to Wilmore, the decrease in resting heart rate that can be expected due to endurance training is one beat per minute each week for the first few weeks of training.[10] Additional cardiorespiratory adaptations lead to, "structural remodeling that improves vascularization of the myocardium", including an increase in coronary perfusion and capillarization.[10,15]

McArdle believes the increase in cardiac output is primarily responsible for significant changes in performance. Other researchers argue a combination of central and peripheral adaptations leads to increased function, and others believe the change in the peripheral system has the greatest effect on increased performance.[10-11,17]

The peripheral adaptations that occur lead primarily to an expanded a-vO$_2$ difference.[10-11,17] The ability of the system to extract and utilize more oxygen, specific to the exercising muscles, enables the cardiovascular system to be more efficient. While Pollock found an average increase in maximal oxygen extraction of 20% in untrained subjects following participation in a six-month training program, McArdle found an average increase of 11% following eight weeks of training.[11,18]

The peripheral vasculature undergoes adaptations including an increase in capillary density surrounding each muscle fiber, specific to the exercised muscle, which facilitates an increase in blood flow to the exercised muscle, resulting in increased oxygen delivery. This enables regional blood flow to increase up to 60%.[10-11,15,19-20]

The redirection of blood flow or shunting of blood to the working muscles increases with endurance training.[10-11,15,19-20] The increased blood flow and perfusion to the working muscle increases the amount of oxygen delivery and transport into the muscle.[10-11,15,17] The concentration of muscle myoglobin has been shown to increase and remain unchanged and hemoglobin concentrations have been shown to increase.[10,15,20] Myoglobin transports oxygen molecules from the cell membrane to the mitochondria and hemoglobin transports oxygen in the blood. Blood volume and the number of red blood cells increases as a result of endurance training leading to a reduced blood viscosity.[10] The reduction in viscosity allows an increase in blood flow, especially to the capillaries, which may also increase performance. This, however, may lead to pseudoanemia, or a corresponding decrease in hematocrit due to the increase in plasma volume.[10]

Exercise induces metabolic adaptations that alter blood lipid levels. Haskell suggests that the enzymes responsible for triglyceride and cholesterol synthesis, transport, and catabolism most likely mediate the exercise-induced changes in lipid and lipoprotein metabolism.[21] While lower triglyceride levels and LDL cholesterol levels have been found in physically active versus inactive adults, Bouchard found that regular physical activity lowers plasma triglycerides in subjects with initially high levels but has little impact on those with normal concentrations.[5,16,22] With physical activity, numerous studies have documented decreases in LDL cholesterol[14,21,23-30] and total cholesterol,[14,21,24,29] while other studies document no change in total cholesterol and LDL cholesterol levels.[22,27,31] In the studies analyzing alterations in serum lipid and triglyceride levels, however, it is unclear whether nutritional intervention was incorporated into the exercise program. According to Stefanick, when beneficial HDL cholesterol or triglyceride changes are reported, the training period is usually at least 12 weeks in length and is often accompanied by significant fat weight loss.[22] Methodological differences in the studies analyzing the effects of exercise on serum lipid and triglyceride values include length of the study, and frequency, intensity and duration of the exercise intervention as well as diet composition.[22]

Increased levels of HDL cholesterol have been documented in physically active people;[5,21-22,25,31] however, research studies have found conflicting evidence of alterations in HDL cholesterol when measured prior to and after participation in an exercise intervention program.[21,32-35] Bouchard suggests a general increase in HDL levels following participation in exercise programs, and proposes the activity of lipoprotein lipase contributes to the augmentation of the HDL cholesterol level.[16] He also postulates that the reduction of hepatic lipase activity as observed with active individuals may play a role in increased HDL cholesterol levels. Physical activity also affects insulin action, as activity appears to mimic an insulin response in peripheral tissues by increasing insulin sensitivity and reducing plasma insulin levels.[16] These mechanisms also may play a role and contribute to alterations in plasma lipid levels following participation in exercise programs.

Alterations in lipoprotein subfractions may account for variance in measured total lipoprotein levels. The consequential decrease in total serum cholesterol may be mediated by a combination of a reduction in LDL cholesterol and a subsequent increase in HDL cholesterol, leading to a reduced change in total serum cholesterol levels.[21,25] Concurrently, a significant reduction in total cholesterol may induce a slight reduction in HDL cholesterol. There appears to be a lack of consensus in the literature regarding the effects of exercise on lipid subfractions. There also appears to be a lack of research evidence that has investigated the relationship between the changes in serum lipids and other physiological variables.

The leading contributor to premature morbidity and mortality in essential hypertensives is CHD. Physical activity is a nonpharmacological treatment that is often featured prominently in the treatment of essential hypertension and used in the primary prevention of hypertension.[11,36] The hemodynamic mechanism whereby exercise reduces total peripheral resistance is unclear. It is believed that a reduction in sympathetic nervous system activity plays a significant role.[10-11,36] While cardiac output and peripheral vascular resistance have been shown to be reduced with equal frequency, researchers postulate that the interaction of the renin-angiotensin-aldosterone system (increased sodium excretion and decreased blood and plasma volume) also plays a role.[11,36]

Hagberg analyzed 47 studies on the effects of exercise intervention in subjects with essential hypertension.[36] Seventy percent of the groups in the studies experienced significant decreases in systolic blood pressure (SBP) and 78% of the groups experienced a reduction in diastolic blood pressure (DBP). The mean reduction in SBP was 10.5 mmHg from an initial level of 154 mmHg. DBP reduced 8.6 mmHg from an initial value of 98 mmHg. This reduction is consistent with research studies as reported by the American College of Sports Medicine.[11] Wilmore adds that exercise intervention is beneficial in mild to moderate hypertensives, but has little effect on people with severe hypertension.[10] McArdle states that the effects of exercise training on blood pressure are most apparent in patients with mild hypertension.[11]

Active individuals have lower SBP and DBP readings than inactive adults and are at a reduced risk of developing hypertension.[5,10-11,36] In normotensive individuals, systolic and diastolic blood pressure can be expected to decrease from 6-10 mmHg with regular aerobic exercise.[11]

Other health benefits are experienced when exercise programs are designed for people with hypertension. Hagberg notes that exercise training increases HDL cholesterol and decreases the ratio of total cholesterol to HDL cholesterol in hypertensives.[36] Exercise training also appears to reduce insulin levels and improve insulin sensitivity and glucose tolerance in hypertensives, therefore, reducing risks associated with other CVD primary risk factors.[10-11]

Obesity, body fat and weight control are critical public health issues as almost two out of every three (61%) of all Americans are either overweight or obese.[37] Research has indicated that almost two out of every three Americans, or about 66%, do not get enough exercise, and one out of every four, or 25%, do not exercise at all. The physiological consequences of inactivity are evident in the increased prevalence of chronic diseases including type 2 diabetes, hypertension, obesity, and subsequently CVD. The physiological, biochemical, and molecular adaptations and mechanisms employed to produce elite human performance, for example, enhancements in carbohydrate and lipid metabolism, are the same mechanisms, when not engaged, can be the principal contributors underlying premature chronic disease.

DiPietro completed an in-depth analysis of the effects of exercise on the reduction of weight and body fat. In the inquiry, she examined several comprehensive review articles and two meta-analyses. From the evaluation, the author concluded the following: (a) physical activity affects body composition and weight favorably by promoting fat loss while preserving lean mass; (b) a clear dose-response relationship is evident, people who exercised longer and more often (per session and per program) experienced an increased rate of weight loss; and (c) exercise combined with diet intervention, albeit a slower process, may be a more effective strategy for long term weight regulation.[38]

The mechanisms whereby exercise induces utilization of fat stores in adipose tissue has been studied and reviewed. During exercise the body prefers to utilize triglycerides for fuel and spare the more limited glycogen stores.[10] Exercise intensity is one of the prime factors related to substrate metabolism; during lower intensity activity a higher percentage of lipids or free fatty acid (FFA) will be oxidized and during higher intensity exercise a larger percentage of carbohydrate stores will be used.[39] Substrate metabolism and its relationship to exercise intensity will be extensively reviewed in the following chapter.

REFERENCES

1. Blair, S.N., Kohl III, H.W., Paffenberger, R.S., Clark, G.G., Cooper, K.H., & Gibbons, L.W. (1989). "Physical fitness and all-cause mortality." *Journal of the American Medical Association* 262, 2395-2401.

2. Paffenberger, R.S., & Hale, W.E. (1975). "Work activity and coronary heart mortality." *New England Journal of Medicine* 292, 545-550.

3. Haskell, W.L. (1994). "Sedentary lifestyle as a risk factor for coronary heart disease." In T.A. Pearson, M.H. Criqui, R.K. Luepker, A. Oberman, & M. Winston (Eds.), *AHA Primer in Preventive Cardiology.* (pp. 173-188). Dallas: American Heart Association.

4. Price, S.A., & Wilson, L.M. (1992). *Pathophysiology: Clinical Concepts of Disease Process.* (4th ed., pp. 81-83). St. Louis: Mosby.

5. Orr, N., Dooly, C. (1999). "The effects of chronic physical activity on the health and fitness profiles of adults". *Medicine and Science in Sport and Exercise* 31(5)134.

6. Pauley, J.T., Palmer, J.A., Wright, C.C., & Pfeiffer, G.J. (1982). "The effect of a 14 week employee wellness program on selected physiological parameters". *Journal of Occupational Medicine* 24, 457-463.

7. Centers for Disease Control and Prevention. (1993). "Public health focus: Physical activity and the prevention of coronary heart disease." *Morbidity Mortality Weekly Report*, 42, 669-672.

8. Kemmer, F.W., & Berger, M. (1983). "Exercise and diabetes mellitus: Physical activity as part of daily life and its role in the treatment of diabetic patients." *International Journal of Sports Medicine* 4, 77-88.

9. Seals, D.R., & Hagberg, J.M. (1984). "The effect of exercise training on human hypertension: a review." *Medicine and Science in Sports and Exercise* 16, 207-215.

10. Wilmore, J.H., & Costill, D.L. (1994). *Physiology of Sport and Exercise.* (p. 289). Champaign: Human Kinetics.

11. McArdle, W.D., Katch, F.I., & Katch, V.L. (2001). *Exercise Physiology: Energy, Nutrition, and Human Performance* (5th ed., pp. 344-345, 922-924). Boston: Williams and Wilkins.

12. American College of Sports Medicine. (1995). *Guidelines for Exercise Testing and Prescription.* (5th ed., p. 156). Baltimore: Williams and Wilkins.

13. Orr, N. (1997). "Effects of a Health Promotion Program on Select Cardiovascular Risk Factors", *American Journal of Health Promotion* 11(6)445.

14. Orr, N., Dooly, C. (2001). "The Effects of Exercise Duration on Cardiovascular Disease Risk Factors: A Comparison of Two Groups", *Medicine and Science in Sport and Exercise* 33(5)4.

15. Booth, F.W., & Thompson, D.B. (1991). "Molecular and cellular adaptation of muscle in response to exercise: Perspectives of various models." *Physiological Reviews* 71, 547-559, 566-573.

16. Bouchard, C. (1995). "Overview of the biological and physiological mechanisms by which different forms of physical activity prevent cardiovascular disease." NIH Consensus Development Conference Abstract, 37-40.

17. Holloszy, J.O. & Coyle, E.F. (1984). "Adaptations of skeletal muscle to endurance exercise and their metabolic consequences." *Journal of Applied Physiology* 56, 831-8.

18. Pollock, M.L., & Wilmore, J.H. (1990). *Exercise in Health and Disease: Evaluation and Prescription for Prevention and Rehabilitation* (2nd ed.). Philadelphia: Saunders.

19. Armstrong, R.B. (1979). "Biochemistry: Energy liberation and use." In R.H. Strauss (Ed.). *Sports Medicine and Physiology.* (pp. 3-28). Philadelphia: Saunders.

20. Hultman, E. (1988). "Carbohydrate metabolism: Principles of exercise biochemistry." *Medicine and Science in Sports and Exercise* 27, 78-119.

21. Haskell, W.L. (1984). "Exercise-induced changes in plasma lipids and lipoproteins." *Preventative Medicine* 13, 23.

22. Stefanick, M.L. (1994). "Exercise, lipoproteins, and cardiovascular disease." In G. F. Fletcher (Ed.), *Cardiovascular Response to Exercise* (pp. 325-345). Mount Krisco: Futura Publishing Co. Inc.

23. Durstine, J.L., & Haskell, W.A. (1994). "Effect of exercise training on plasma lipids and lipoproteins." *Exercise and Sport Science Reviews* 24, 477-500.

24. Goldberg, L., Elliot, D.L, & Schultz, R.W. (1984). "Changes in lipid lipoprotein levels after weight training." *Journal of the American Medical Association* 225,504.

25. Hurley, B.F., Seals, D.R., & Hagberg, J.M. (1984). "High-density-lipoprotein cholesterol in bodybuilders versus powerlifters: Negative effects of androgen use." *Journal of the American Medical Association* 254, 507.

26. Krummel, D., Etherton, T.D., Peterson, S., & Kris-Etherton, P.M. (1993). "Effects of exercise on plasma lipids and lipoproteins of women." PSEBM, 240, 123-37.

27. Stefanick, M.L. (1995). "Physical activity and lipid metabolism." NIH Consensus Development Conference Abstract, 65-67.

28. Williams, P.T., Wood, P.D., & Haskell, W.L. (1982). "The effects of running mileage and duration on plasma lipoprotein levels." *Journal of the American Medical Association* 2674.

29. Cyr, N. (2002). "Intervention Strategies to Improve Blood Lipid Levels." *American Journal of Health Promotion* 16(6)361-2.

30. Orr, N. (1997). "Effects of Nutrition Intervention on Serum Cholesterol Levels." *American Journal of Health Promotion* 11(6)446.

31. Durstine, J.L., & Haskell, W.A. (1994). "Effect of exercise training on plasma lipids and lipoproteins." *Exercise and Sport Science Reviews* 24, 501-521.

32. Cook, T.C., Laprote, R.E., & Washburn, R.A. (1986). "Chronic low level physical activity as a determinant of high density lipoprotein cholesterol and subfractions." *Medicine and Science in Sports and Exercise* 18, 653.

33. Gaesser, G.A., & Rich, R.G. (1984). "Effects of high-and low-intensity exercise training on aerobic capacity and blood lipids." *Medicine and Science in Sports and Exercise* 16, 269.

34. Goldberg, L., & Elliot, D.L. (1985). "The effect of physical activity on lipid and lipoprotein levels." *Medical Clinic North American* 69, 41.

35. Orr, N., Dooly, C. (2000). "The Effects of a University Based Employee Health Promotion Program on Cardiovascular Risk Profiles". *Medicine and Science in Sport and Exercise* 32(5)126.

36. Hagberg, J.M. (1995). "Physical activity, physical fitness, and blood pressure." *NIH Consensus Development Conference Abstract*, 69-71.

37. Nieman, D.C. (2003). *Exercise Testing and Prescription a Health Related Approach.* (pp. 508-522). New York, NY: McGraw-Hill Higher Education.

38. DiPietro, L. (1995). "Physical activity, body weight, and adiposity. An epidemiologic perspective." *Exercise and Sport Science Reviews* 27, 281-296.

39. Bulow, J. (1988). "Lipid mobilization and utilization: Principles of exercise biochemistry." *Medicine and Science in Sports and Exercise* 20, 140-163.

CHAPTER FIVE

EXERCISE BIOCHEMISTRY

This chapter introduces exercise biochemistry and provides an extensive analysis of the biochemical adaptations that occur in response to exercise and physical activity.

The extent and level of substrate metabolism is dependent upon exercise intensity (Figure 5.1). Throughout a two-hour exercise session, the percentages remain relatively constant and the predominant substrates remain muscle glycogen, plasma free-fatty acids, and muscle triglycerides. When exercise intensity is reduced to 25% VO_2 max., the predominant substrate used is plasma free-fatty acids (up to 90%).

This research helps support the argument of prescribing lower intensity exercise sessions to facilitate fat loss in an exercise intervention program. The other factors related to substrate metabolism are diet (substrate availability), an individuals overall health status, and state of physical training.[1]

Triglycerides are stored mainly in adipose tissue, but are also stored within the muscle, and are available from circulating lipoproteins (FFA). Liver stores of triglycerides are not utilized

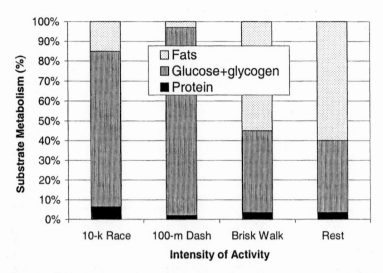

FIGURE 5.1 – The relationship between exercise intensity and substrate metabolism.

during exercise and the greatest amount of stored energy is located in adipose tissue. The rate controlling enzyme of lipid metabolism is hormone sensitive lipase (HSL), which facilitates the degradation of triacylglycerides to diacylglycerol and to monoacylglycerol.[2]

Circulating lipoproteins are catalyzed by lipoprotein lipase (LPL), which is widely distributed in the body (the highest concentrations are found in the heart, adipose tissue and slow twitch red skeletal muscle). LPL is synthesized within the cell and transported to the surface of the capillary endothelium. The enzyme activity of LPL is dependent on the need for lipid storage or lipid mobilization. Adrenaline and noradrenaline are the main lipolytic hormones, and insulin is the only antilipolytic hormone. A certain amount of LPL remains in the muscle to facilitate intramuscular triacylglyceride breakdown. The mechanisms responsible for increased lipolysis are sympathoadrenal activity and decreased insulin levels. Thyroid function (specifically thyroxin and TDH) may also play a part in lipolysis.[2]

The body either stores triacylglycerides (re-esterification) or breaks them down (lipolysis), and this capacity is determined by the amount of albumin (carrier of FFA in the blood), blood flow and the number of binding sites occupied (arterial FFA/albumin ratio). About two-thirds of the fatty acids liberated by lipolysis during exercise are re-esterified. While high FFA/albumin ratios will retard lipolysis and blood lactate enhances lipid re-esterification, during long duration activities, blood FFA concentrations stabilize.[2]

Physical activity or endurance training results in an increased sensitivity to insulin because exercise has an insulin like effect on skeletal muscle; it increases the sensitivity in the β–adrenergic agonists without an increase in the number of receptors. Consequentially, participation in exercise programs results in an increased lipid mobilization capacity and an increased ability to replenish triacylglycerol stores.[2]

Free fatty acids, attached to albumin, are transported in the blood and pass into the cell where they are converted to acyl-CoA and either re-esterified (stored) or β-oxidized (broken down and utilized). Predominantly slow-twitch red fibers oxidize FFA during moderate intensity exercise. Carnitine is the enzyme responsible for the transport of acyl-CoA from the cytoplasm into the mitochondria matrix. Carnitine is either synthesized (75%) or ingested and it is actively transported into the cell. If carnitine is not available abnormalities in lipid metabolism will occur. Two main factors regulate FFA oxidation, the availability of FFA as determined by FFA mobilization and the capacity of the tissues to oxidize FFA. Ketone bodies are a very small contributor (<7%) to exercise metabolism and are usually spared for nonmuscular tissues, such as the brain.[2]

Transferring the biochemical and physiological adaptations to decreased incidence of chronic disease, Blair analyzed studies investigating the relationship between physical activity and physical fitness and selected chronic diseases over a thirty-year time-period. The most substantial findings were a significant decrease in all-cause mortality and coronary artery disease. Additional significant results indicated a decrease in hypertension, obesity, certain types of cancer, type 2 diabetes, osteoporosis, and significant increases in functional capacity.[3]

Participation in exercise programs may also induce changes in physiological parameters that may alter performance variables. Included in these changes are an increase in mitochondria and capillary density. The increases in mitochondria and capillary density are specific to muscle fiber recruited for the activity, and are specific to the muscle fiber type.[4-5] Muscle fibers have been subdivided into two main classifications, type I and type II with type II fibers subdivided into type II^a and type II^b. Type I or slow oxidative red fibers contain five to six capillaries per muscle fiber; type II^a or fast oxidative glycolytic red contain four capillaries per muscle; and, type II^b or fast glycolytic white contain three capillaries per muscle fiber. On average, a person will have between 45-55% type I fibers which are indicative of endurance athletes and the remaining fibers will consist of type II fibers which are indicative of sprinters/explosive power athletes.[1,5] Although type I fibers have twice the mitochondrial content of type II fibers, the mitochondrial content of type II^b fibers has been shown to increase up to three to four fold following very strenuous endurance training or interval training.[5-6]

While some researchers believe fiber types do not convert as a result of endurance training[4-5,7], others cite research studies that suggest an actual conversion of fiber type when chronic and specific types of activity are employed.[1,8] Type II fibers have been shown to adopt the mechanical or contractile properties or characteristics of type I fibers during certain endurance type activities.[1,7-8]

Along with central (cardiorespiratory) and vascular changes that affect oxygen delivery and extraction, intramuscular adaptations occur to facilitate an increase in performance and measured VO$_2$ max. Adenosine triphosphate (ATP) is produced within the mitochondria of a muscle cell and its synthesis is the rate-limiting factor of carbohydrate oxidation. A chronic adaptation of endurance activity is an increase in the size and number of mitochondria, which results in a subsequent increase in the respiratory capacity of the cell.[1,5-9] Holloszy stated that the protein content of the mitochondria may increase up to 60%, Wilmore documented an increase in size of 35%, and Holloszy determined that total mitochondria may increase four fold.[5,7] Mitochondrial enzymes including creatine kinase, adenylate kinase, α-glycerophosphate dehydrogenase do not increase in response to endurance training.[5] The first enzyme to increase appears to be δ-aminolevulinic acid synthase which is the rate limiting enzyme in heme synthesis.[5,8,10]

The increase in the size and number of the mitochondria permits a lower percentage increase of adenosine diphosphate (ADP) and phosphate (Pi) in each mitochondria during exercise. Restated, the increase in ADP and Pi concentration is dissipated or "spread out" enabling the system to become more efficient.[7,11] This lowers the overall change in the concentration of ADP and Pi. This results in a more efficient flux of glucose into the cell to meet the energy needs of the mitochondria to use pyruvate as fuel for oxidation. The more efficient changes in the ATP/ADP ratio, the less active phosophfructokinase (PFK) would be since ATP and [H+] inhibit PFK.[5,9-10] Since ATP formation equals ATP utilization a metabolic fine tuning occurs which results in a more efficient process. These adaptations lead to an increase in the amount of time a person can exercise until exhaustion and also increases the intensity level at which a person can exercise, therefore, leading to an overall increased work capacity.[5,11]

An increase in the number of enzymes responsible for oxidative phosphorylation which increases the cell's ability to oxidize both pyruvate and fatty acids is another adaptation of endurance training.[1,5,7,11] The enzymes of the tricarboxylic acid (TCA) cycle and the mitochondrial respiratory chain including citrate synthetase and succinate dehydrogenase, nicotinamide adenine dinucleotide (NADH) dehydrogenase, cytochrome *c* reductase, and cytochromoxidase have been shown to increase from at least two fold[5-6,8] to between three and four fold.[7,11]

The oxidative enzymes determine the theoretical maximum rate of substrate or fuel metabolism; since the rate-limiting factor for substrate metabolism is the availability of the enzymes concerned with its metabolism.[9] Therefore, an increase in the number of oxidative enzymes results in an increased capacity to metabolize substrates, which equals an increase in the production of adenosine triphosphate (ATP).[1,5-7] Further exercise-induced adaptations include minor changes and an overall decrease in glycolytic enzymes, except hexokinase.[5,9,11] Evidence of the change in glycolytic enzymes is conflicting.[8,9,11] A review of the literature documents glycogen phosphorylase (the enzyme responsible for glycogen degradation) decreases, increases and remains unchanged. Whereas the debranching enzyme (the enzyme responsible for glycogen resynthesis) has been shown to increase, Booth states that the decrease in glycolytic enzymes is specific to fast-twitch red muscles.[8-9] The adaptations occurring to the mitochondrial enzymes may be more responsive to increased synthesis, rather than decreased degradation, or may result from a combination of both processes.[5,8] Phosphofructokinase (PFK), which dictates the overall rate of glycolytic flux to pyruvate, has been shown to decrease or remain unchanged with endurance activity.[9] Lactate dehydrogenase (LDH), the enzyme responsible for the conversion of lactate to pyruvate decreases with training possibly due to an increase in heart specific LDH-I form.[5,8-10]

An increase in the capacity of the mitochondria to oxidize NADH will also lower the formation of lactate because pyruvate is formed instead of lactate.[9-11] Of the two shuttle mechanisms responsible for trans-mitochondrial membrane transfer of NADH, the glycerol 3-phosphate, and malate-aspirate, the malate-aspirate shuttle mechanism activity increases with endurance training.[5,9] When lactate is not removed from the muscle, the amount of ATP that can be synthesized through the formation of lactate is reduced to 60-75 mMol/kg.[9]

Exercise intervention has been shown to lead to an increased lactate threshold, a decrease in lactate formation (concentration) with higher intensity activities, or a decreased lactate formation at a given rate of glycolysis which corresponds to a decreased lactate dehydrogenase concentration.[5,7,9,12] Additional adaptations include an increase in transporters, co-transporters, and facilitators of muscular contraction, and a possible decrease buildup in the concentration of NH_3 in the blood, with increasing exercise intensity levels.[5,8] The buffering capacity of the exercised muscle is increased through subsequent increases in mitochondrial competition with lactate dehydrogenase for pyruvate.[5,9] This results in an increased intensity level until lactate is formed which leads to a subsequent reduction in the availability of pyruvate to the lactate dehydrogenase system.[5]

Another adaptation from participating in endurance activities is an increased ability of the body to utilize fat as a fuel source in higher intensity activity which results in a decrease in the amount of glycogen used during activity or glycogen sparing.[5,11] This can be quantified through a decreased respiratory quotient (RQ) or respiratory equivalent ratio (RER) at absolute and relative submaximal rates of work.[5,7,11] This alteration in the metabolic response to exercise is in part brought about by smaller changes in ATP and ADP in muscles during exercise and training, which is related to an increased concentration of mitochondria, specific to the trained muscle fibers.[11] This helps maintain adequate ratios of ATP/ADP/AMP/Pi, by increasing the ability of the muscle to translocate ADP into the mitochondria. Ultimately the availability of oxygen is the rate limiting factor in ATP production, however, when sufficient oxygen and substrate are available, the concentration of ADP is the primary factor regulating mitochondrial respiration.[5,9-11]

Increased fatty acid oxidation will increase the citric acid content in the cytoplasm, this will increase the inhibition of PFK, since PFK is activated when the cell needs energy, and inhibited when the cell has enough energy.[9,10] This will lead to an increased concentration of glucose 6-phosphate, which inhibits hexokinase and similarly affects phosphorylase b.[2,9-11]

During prolonged exercise, depending on duration and intensity, glycogen degradation is approximately 2-4 mMol/min (liver weight 1.8 kg) and total liver storage is 160-800 mMol, with a range of 50-900 mMol depending on diet manipulation.[9] Total skeletal and liver stores equal about 2,000 Kcal, resulting in liver glycogen depletion after 1-3 hours of heavy activity or about 20 miles of running.[7,9] Diet manipulation through increased carbohydrate (CHO) ingestion and glycogen depletion exercise, or in the highly trained individual, high CHO diets with decreased activity, can affect glycogen storage, which then can affect endurance capacity.[9] Increased fat utilization and decreased glucose utilization with increasing intensity levels, along with increased intramuscular triacylglyceride storage and increased muscle glycogen stores will increase exercise capacity and increase exercise endurance ability.[5,7]

Better coordination of fat and carbohydrate metabolism is accomplished via changes in the citric acid concentration in the mitochondria and then in the cytoplasm, and through changes in the acetyl coenzyme A (CoA)/CoA ratios.[2,9] An increased ratio of acetyl CoA/CoA will decrease the activity of pyruvate dehydrogenase (PDH) since PDH is inhibited by ATP and stimulated by ADP and AMP.[2,9-10,13]

Another metabolic adaptation related to participation in endurance activities is improved glucose tolerance. The sensitivity of the liver, skeletal muscle, and adipose tissue leads to an increased sensitivity to insulin.[2,14-15] This could be due to the increased number of insulin receptors on the cell's surface, which in turn facilitates increased transport and cellular uptake of glucose for utilization and storage or an increase rate of hepatic removal of insulin or a combination of these mechanisms.[14]

Endurance activities have been related to increased albumin concentrations and an increased capacity to oxidize ketones.[5,7] Albumin is a protein that carries fatty acids from adipose tissue to the muscle cell for degradation. Increases in the enzymes responsible for the activation, transport (albumin), and β-oxidation of long-chain fatty acids have also been determined as well as an increase in mitochondria coupling factor I, resulting in an increased VO_2 max and increased endurance at submaximal VO_2 levels.[5,11]

The adaptations resulting from participation in an endurance activity are specific to the exercised muscle, muscle group, and muscle fiber.[5,16-17] The adaptations require a training stimulus that exceeds the capacity of the muscle, it must be progressively increased to allow additional adaptations to occur.[5] The extent of the adaptations will further increase when the initial conditioning level is low and the adaptations will decrease less in athletes who have been performing for a longer period of time.[5,7]

REFERENCES

1. McArdle, W.D., Katch, F.I., & Katch, V.L. (2001). *Exercise Physiology: Energy, Nutrition, and Human Performance.* (5th ed., pp. 532-534). Boston: Williams and Wilkins.

2. Bulow, J. (1988). "Lipid mobilization and utilization: Principles of exercise biochemistry." *Medicine and Science in Sports and Exercise* 20, 140-163.

3. Blair, S. & McCloy, C.H. (1993). "Research lecture: Physical activity, physical fitness, and health." *Research Quarterly in Exercise*, 64, 365-376.

4. Fitts, R.H., & Widrick, J.J. (1996). "Muscle mechanics: Adaptations with exercise training." *Exercise and Sport Science Reviews* 28, 427-473.

5. Holloszy, J.O. & Coyle, E.F. (1984). "Adaptations of skeletal muscle to endurance exercise and their metabolic consequences." *Journal of Applied Physiology* 56, 831-8.

6. Essig, D.A., (1996). "Contractile activity-induced mitochondrial biogenesis in skeletal muscle." *Exercise and Sport Science Reviews* 28, 289-319.

7. Wilmore, J.H., & Costill, D.L. (1994). *Physiology of Sport and Exercise.* (pp. 222-239). Champaign: Human Kinetics.

8. Booth, F.W., & Thompson, D.B. (1991). "Molecular and cellular adaptation of muscle in response to exercise: Perspectives of various models." *Physiological Reviews* 71, 547-559, 566-573.

9. Hultman, E. (1988). "Carbohydrate metabolism: Principles of exercise biochemistry." *Medicine and Science in Sports and Exercise* 27, 78-119.

10. Southerland, W. M. (1990). *Foundations of medicine: Biochemistry.* (pp. 94-95). New York: Churchill Livingstone.

11. Holloszy, J.O. (1973). "Biochemical adaptations to exercise: Aerobic metabolism." *Exercise and Sports Science Reviews* 1, 45-71.

12. Armstrong, R.B. (1979). "Biochemistry: Energy liberation and use." In R. H. Strauss (Ed.), *Sports Medicine and Physiology.* (pp. 3-28). Philadelphia: Saunders.

13. Duan, C., & Winder, W. (1994). "Effect of endurance training on activators of glycolysis in muscle during exercise." *American Physiological Society*, 846-852.

14. Constn-Teodosiu, D. (1991). "Acetyl group accumulation and pyruvate dehydrogenase activity in human muscle during incremental exercise." *Acta Physiol Scand*, 143, 367-372.

15. Bouchard, C. (1995). "Overview of the biological and physiological mechanisms by which different forms of physical activity prevent cardiovascular disease." NIH Consensus Development Conference Abstract, 37-40.

16. Gulve, E.A. (1992). "Effects of acute and chronic exercise on insulin-stimulated glucose transport activity in skeletal muscle." *Medicine and Science in Sports and Exercise* 24, 273-280.

17. Fitts, R.H., & Widrick, J.J. (1996). "Muscle mechanics: Adaptations with exercise training." *Exercise and Sport Science Reviews* 28, 427-473.

CHAPTER SIX

EFFICACY OF HEALTH PROMOTION PROGRAMS

This chapter provides the historical and theoretical framework and chronicles the evolution of wellness and employer sponsored health promotion programs. It presents valuable information on program components, documents efficacy, and includes return on investment (ROI) data.

Since a high proportion of the American population is employed, the worksite setting offers immense potential for the implementation of health promotion programs.[1] The potential for behavioral change is evident as the workplace offers opportunities to make repeated contacts with large and diverse groups of individuals, follow-up is easier than in clinical or community-based programs, and worksites have already existing social support systems for behavioral changes.[2] Two of the pioneers in comprehensive employee health promotion programs include Johnson & Johnson's Live for Life program begun in 1979 and Campbell Soup Company's Turnaround Health and Fitness Program initiated in 1982.[3-4] Both of these programs exemplified a comprehensive approach to health promotion addressing behavioral, preventive, and environmental aspects of employee health enhancement. While Johnson & Johnson and Campbells are recognized as being leaders in comprehensive programming, corporations have been concerned about their employees health since the 1920s. Health screening, employee assistance, and health education promoted a decrease in infectious diseases, and assistance to employees for personal problems were common throughout the 1950s. Although these programs did give educational materials to employees, they usually did not provide time, space, or change of worksite routine, nor was there a genuine commitment from top management.[5]

Although the first published report of health education in worksite settings was a 1957 survey of the Massachusetts area plants, health education activities were provided by community agencies and consisted mainly of dispersing information concerning the availability of community-based programs.[6] These early programs, nominally referred to as health education, are accurately depicted as marketing ploys by community health agencies such as the American Heart Association, American Cancer Association, and other similar organizations. These programs were not popular with workers or management because the prevailing concerns of both groups revolved mainly around reduction of industrial safety hazards. Interventions designed by agencies committed to improving specific aspects of public health such as those listed earlier unsurprisingly were ill-equipped to effectively design programs to adequately meet the perceived needs to their target population.[7]

Employer interest in sponsoring health promotion activities started to emerge in the mid-1970s and when in 1980 the U.S. Department of Health and Human Services published the 1990 Health Objectives for the Nation, health promotion programs seemed to be as firmly established in the workplace as in other sites.[8] The growth in worksite programs has partly resulted from the belief that an organization should assume a certain level of responsibility for the health of its most valued resource, the employee.[5]

The Health Wise Stepped Intervention study (1988-1990) at Pacific Gas and Electric was an evaluation of the effects of a health promotion program on behavior change and was initiated to determine whether implementation of preventive interventions improved health status. Physiological measurements of weight, blood pressure, total serum cholesterol, and HDL cholesterol were assessed in 4,164 employees. The results of this study showed an overall reduction in risk factors as all four physiological parameters improved.[9]

According to the Wellness Councils of America, worksite health promotion programs increase productivity, improve morale, reduce turnover and absenteeism, and improve public relations.[10] While companies recognize the social and physical benefits of implementing health promotion programs, containment of health care costs is the primary reason given by employers for implementing a program.[11]

Many companies have reported considerable savings in health-related costs resulting from health promotion programs.[12-13] A study by Health Promotion Services, a Blue Cross of Western Pennsylvania affiliate, reported a positive relationship between participation in a health promotion program, health care utilization, and cost control.[14] Stead reported that for every dollar that Coors Brewing Company invests in wellness activities, a return savings of over six dollars is realized. Annually, Coors reports a savings of $1.9 million through reduced medical costs, sick leave, and increased productivity.[15]

The Jaynes Corporation, which has 200-300 employees, provides another example in health care cost reduction through worksite health promotion. In this study, a 20% reduction in health care premiums were reported.[16] Povell, reported an overall cost-savings ratio of 3:1, or for every dollar invested, three dollars are saved.[17]

While the large majority (67%) of employee wellness programs are paid for and administered by the company, the savings are not limited to an individual corporation, or a state, as insurance carriers are beginning to recognize the financial impact of employee wellness programs. Roush found that several major insurers, including Metropolitan Life, Prudential, John Hancock, Travelers, and Aetna are reducing group life premiums for the companies that offer some type of wellness program.[18]

A majority of business concerns arise from increasing health care costs and the possibility of impending government regulations such as universal coverage and mandates for employer provided health insurance for all employees. During the past ten years, the cost of providing employee medical benefits increased more than twice the rate of inflation. According to Harvey, in 1980 the national average cost per employee for medical benefits was $968, compared to $1,740 per employee in 1985, and $3,250 per employee in 1990.[19] Since the last decade, health care costs have risen. In 2001, the net cost of private health insurance increased 11.2%, and the projected annual increase for 2004-2008 is 6.2%. According to Stead, business was responsible for 17% of the total U.S. medical bill in 1973, and by 1993 the percentage had increased to approximately 30%.[15] Estimations of the proportion of employee health care costs paid for by employers range from 28% to over one-third of acquired expenses. Clearly, the implementation of employer sponsored wellness programs is one strategy used by companies to help control and relieve the economic burden of health care costs.

In 1985, the National Survey of Worksite Health Promotion Activities was used to determine the extent of worksite wellness activities. Priority areas from Healthy People were used as guidelines for the collection of baseline data important in assessing both quantity and quality of worksite health enhancement programs.[20] Over 1,635 worksites having 50 or more employees were surveyed, with 65% having at least one health promotion activity provided for their employees. The leading activities were smoking cessation programs/policies, physical activity/fitness activities, hypertension/ hypercholesterolemia education/screenings. This study was reinforced when Fielding reported that two-thirds of all worksites of similar size had some kind of health promotion program.[21]

In 1992, replication of the National Survey of Worksite Health Promotion Activities study included 1,507 worksites and found that 81% of employers had at least one health promotion activity. Differences and increases were noted in comparison to 1985 in terms of prevalence of activities offered in all measured areas including hypertension and hypercholesterolemia education/ screenings, physical activity/fitness programs, smoking cessation programs and policies, nutrition education, weight control, stress management, cancer, safety, and alcohol/drug education. McGinnis graphed a comparison of the data from the 1985 and 1992 surveys, along with the goals of Healthy People 2000.[22] In the analysis, the author reported percent increases from 1985-1992 in the following areas: physical activity/fitness-54% to 83%, nutrition education-17% to 31%, weight control programs-15% to 24%, hypertension/hypercholesterolemia programs/screenings-17% to 35%. While the totals remained below the objectives of Healthy People 2000, the increases and progress towards the objectives of Healthy People 2000 were encouraging.

The established goal of 75% of worksites offering employer sponsored physical activity and fitness programs is the designated target listed in Healthy People 2010. In 1999, 46% of worksites with 50 or more employees offered physical activity and/or fitness programs at the worksite or through their health plans. This percentage seems to increase as the size of the company increases, with 68% of the largest worksites offering programs.

While the rank order of the activities offered remains relatively stable, the prevalence of programming is related to the size of the corporation.[23] Major exceptions to this trend were worksites with fewer than 250 employees, which had more smoking cessation programs than any other type of activity. Also worksites with over 750 employees had more health risk assessment activities, followed by stress management, and smoking. In 1985, the Office of Disease Prevention and Health Promotion conducted a survey to determine the extent of programming based on organization size.[24] Fifty-four percent of companies with 750 or more employees offered exercise/physical fitness programs, 66% offered health risk appraisal inventories, and 61% offered programs on stress management.

According to the 1989 Monthly Vital Statistics Report from the National Center for Health Statistics, each of the ten leading causes of death was associated with some voluntary aspect of lifestyle, such as diet, smoking, inactivity, or excessive alcohol consumption. This report indirectly concluded that wellness and disease prevention intervention has the potential to change unhealthy lifestyle habits, which lead to risk reduction and, therefore, cost containment or reduction. The ten leading causes of death account for 82% of all fatalities in the nation. Seven of the top ten leading causes of death in descending order are cardiovascular disease, cancers, stroke, accident, chronic obstructive lung disease, pneumonia/influenza, and diabetes mellitus.[25] Aside from accidents, all of the leading causes of death can be influenced and affected by minor lifestyle modifications.

The 2001 Monthly Vital Statistics Report from the National Center for Health Statistics lists heart disease as the number one cause of death, followed by cancer, cerebrovascular accidents, chronic lower respiratory diseases, accidents, diabetes mellitus, pneumonia and influenza, alzheimers disease, kidney disease, and septicemia.[26] Heart disease, cancer, and cerebrovascular disease account for over 60% of the total (60.4%), the remaining seven causes account for 39.6% of the total. Research studies have demonstrated that heart disease, certain types of cancer, and cerebrovascular disease may have specific behavioral and lifestyle links subject to modification.

Research studies have demonstrated that these minor lifestyle modifications can be influenced by the implementation of employer sponsored health promotion and wellness programs.[27-32] Briley documented a reduction in total cholesterol levels and weight when nutrition education programs were added to an employee wellness program.[29] In this research, the author found that major changes in blood lipid levels occurred within the first twelve weeks of the study. HDL cholesterol increased throughout the study, most likely due to the combination of increased activity and diet modifications. This research documents the importance of combining exercise intervention with diet modifications.

Cyr found that health promotion programs that incorporate nutrition intervention strategies can significantly reduce total cholesterol, and LDL cholesterol, and improve the ratio of TC:HDL cholesterol.[31]

Aldana researched the effects of employee health promotion programs on a variety of cardiovascular risk factors including blood pressure, percent body fat, submaximal cardiovascular fitness, and blood lipids including total cholesterol (TC), and the ratio of TC to HDL cholesterol.[27] The primary emphasis of the program was to provide extensive pre-participant screening and target specific higher risk characteristics and behaviors with substantial educational information and comprehensive guidance from a variety of health care providers. After taking measurements at baseline, and at 6, 12 and 18 month intervals, the author observed significant changes ($p \leq 0.01$) in all of the physiological variables measured. This research is consistent with research conducted by Cyr that demonstrated a significant improvement in cardiovascular fitness, systolic blood pressure, percent body fat, BMI, body weight, and total cholesterol (TC) after participation in a sixteen week employer sponsored health promotion program.[32]

Fries conducted a longitudinal study to assess the changes in health risks in a community based health promotion program utilizing 103,937 people who were observed for at least six months up to 30 months.[33] Health habit improvements were documented in systolic and diastolic blood pressure, total cholesterol, and exercise time (minutes per week) following the dissemination of educational literature aimed at improving the awareness of health and lifestyle habits. This research supports the importance of the inclusion of educational intervention in improving health habits.

A 2002 survey listed the top eight benefits cited most frequently by worksites offering health promotion programs.[34] They were:

1) 28% - improved employee health
2) 26% - improved employee morale
3) 19% - reduced health insurance cost
4) 19% - reduced absenteeism
5) 16% - increased productivity
6) 9% - reduced accidents on the job
7) 7% - improved education on health issues
8) 4% - reduced workers' compensation claims

Cost, lack of management support, and lack of interested employees were the three most common barriers to implementing employer sponsored health promotion programs.[34]

More recently a collateral focus on the efficacy of health promotion programs has shifted to documenting the cost-effectiveness to employers[13,33,35] and connecting the cost-effectiveness to improvements in work performance and reductions in absenteeism.[36-38] Yen evaluated the association between health risk appraisal scores and medical claim costs and found strong statistical evidence that employees with positive health behaviors cost less in medical claims.[35] Quantifying specific monetary savings, Chapman conducted an extensive cost-effectiveness analysis and concluded an average cost benefit ratio of 1:5.94.[13] Restated, for every dollar an employer invested in a health promotion program, the net savings was almost six dollars.

A comprehensive review, published in 1999, analyzed return on investment (ROI) data from studies on corporate health and productivity management initiatives.[12] The results of this investigation indicate a broad range of return on investment estimates and calculations. This range spanned from a low of $1.49 in benefits per dollar spent to a high of $13. The range was dependent on the type of program offered, and the available data used for analysis. Nine studies were included in the analysis on corporate health management ROIs. The range of benefit-to-cost ratios for these programs was about $1.50-$4.90 in benefits per dollar spent on the program. The median ROI was about $3.14 in benefits per dollar spent. Study participants included in the research evaluations ranged from 517 to 49,249.

Leutzinger published a study that projected future medical care costs based upon the implementation of employer sponsored health promotion programs at Union Pacific Railroad (UPRR).[39] UPRR is a transportation company that employs more than 56,000 employees in 25 states west and south of the Mississippi River. The economic forecasting model investigated the projected increase in medical care costs and considered employee demographics and health risk profiles over a ten year time period. The authors concluded that without health promotion intervention, seven of the 11 risk factors assessed would likely worsen among the UPRR workforce. Medical care costs increases were projected to range from $22.2 million to $99.6 million in constant 1998 dollars over the next decade, dependent on the effectiveness of the risk factor modification program. The model forecasted that with an average health promotion program budget of $1.9 million annually over ten years, health risks must decline at least 0.9% per year for the program to pay for itself. The authors concluded that this type of forecasting model can be used in program planning and help produce an economic justification for the implementation of health promotion programs.

REFERENCES

1. Neiman, D.C. (1995). *Fitness and Sports Medicine: A Health Related Approach*. (3rd ed., p. 22). Palo Alto: Bull.

2. Hartman, T.J., Himes, J.H., McCarthy, P.R. & Kushi, L.H. (1995). "Effects of a low-fat, worksite intervention on blood lipids and lipoproteins." *American College of Occupational and Environmental Medicine* 11, 120-3.

3. Wilbur, C.S. (1983). "The Johnson and Johnson program." *Preventive Medicine* 12, 672-681.

4. Melcalfe, L.L. (1986). "Campbell Soup Company's Turnaround health and fitness program." *American Journal of Health Promotion.*

5. Gebhardt, D.L. & Crump, C.E. (1990). "Employee fitness and wellness programs in the marketplace." *American Psychologist* 45, 262-71.

6. Ware, B. (1982). "Health education in occupational settings: History has its message." *Health Education Quarterly* 9 (supp), 37-41.

7. Hunt, B.P. (1994). "An assessment of the comprehensiveness of health promotion programs included in the 1992 National Survey of Worksite Health Promotion Activities." Unpublished doctoral dissertation, University of Alabama, Tuscaloosa, AL.

8. U.S. Department of Health and Human Services. (1980). "Objectives for the nation 1990." Silver Springs, MD: Office of Disease Prevention and Health Promotion.

9. Shi, L. (1992). "The impact of increasing intensity of health promotion intervention on risk reduction." *Evaluation and the Health Professionals* 15, 3-25.

10. Grobman, M. (1991). "Helping employees stay healthy." *Business & Health* 9, 10-11.

11. Katz, P.P., & Shoestack, J.A. (1990). "Is it worth it? Evaluating the economic impact of worksite health promotion." *Occupational Medicine: State of the Art Reviews* 5, 837-850.

12. Goetzel, R.Z., Juday, T.R., Ozminkowski, R. (1999). "What's The ROI?" *Association of Worksite Health Promotion Worksite Health.* Summer, 12-21.

13. Chapman, L.S. (1995). "Meta-Analysis of Studies on the Cost-Effectiveness of Worksite Health Promotion Programs." Paper presented at the meeting of the American Journal of Health Promotion, Orlando, FL.

14. Papale, M.A. & Lawless, G.D. (1993). "The impact of lifestyle health risk on the bottom line: A case study." *Employee Benefits Journal* 18, 19-21.

15. Stead, B.A. (1994). "Worksite health programs: A significant cost-cutting approach." *Business Horizons* 37, 73-78.

16. Larock, S. (1994). "Does wellness pay? Two employers say "yes"--and prove it." *Employee Benefit Plan Review* 49, 52-62.

17. Povell, J. (1994). "Wellness strategies: How to choose a health risk appraisal." *Compensation and Benefits Review* 26, 59-64.

18. Roush, J. (1994). "Wellness can trim bottom line." *Business Week* 112.

19. Harvey, C.S. (1993). "Making employees partners in the health care purchasing decision." *Employee Benefits Journal* 18, 23.

20. U.S. Department of Health, Education, and Welfare. (1979). *Healthy People: The Surgeon General's Report on Health Promotion and Disease Prevention.* (DHEW Publication No PHS 79-55071). Washington, DC: Government Printing Office.

21. Fielding, J.E., & Pisrchia, P.V. (1989). "Frequency of worksite health promotion activities." *American Journal of Public Health* 79, 16-20.

22. McGinnis, J.M., & Foege, W.H. (1993). "Actual causes of death in the United States." *Journal of American Medication Association* 270, 2207-2212.

23. Fielding, J.E., & Breslow, L. (1983). "Health promotion programs sponsored by California employers." *American Journal of Public Health* 73, 538-542.

24. Thornberry, O.T., Wilson, R.W., & Golden, P.M. (1986). "The 1985 health promotion and disease prevention survey." *The Public Health Reports*, 101, 566-570.

25. U.S. Department of Health and Human Services. (1990). *Healthy People 2000 National Health Promotion and Disease Prevention Objectives.* (DHHS Publication No PHS 91-50213). Washington, DC: Government Printing Office (5)392-395.

26. National Center for Health Statistics (2001). "Monthly Vital Statistics Report." 49(3). Hyattsville, MD.

27. Aldana, S.G., Jacobson, B.H., & Kelley, P.L. (1993). "Mobile work site health promotion program can reduce selected employee health risks." *Journal of Occupational Medicine* 35, 922-928.

28. Baun, B., Williams, L. (1985). "Tenneco: Building corporate quality through good health." *Management Review*, 74, 51-53.

29. Briley, M.E., Montgomery, D.W., & Blewett, J. (1992). "Worksite nutrition education can lower total cholesterol levels and promote weight loss among police department employees." *Journal of the American Dietetic Association* 92, 1372-1384.

30. Erfert, J., et al. (1991). "The cost-effectiveness of work-site wellness programs for hypertension control, weight loss, and smoking cessation." *Journal of Occupational Medicine* 33, 962-970.

31. Cyr, N. (2002). "Intervention Strategies to Improve Blood Lipid Levels." *American Journal of Health Promotion* 16(6)361-2.

32. Orr, N., Dooly, C. (2000). "The Effects of a University Based Employee Health Promotion Program on Cardiovascular Risk Profiles." *Medicine and Science Sport and Exercise* 32(5)126.

33. Fries, J.F., Fries, J.T., Parcell, C.L., & Harrington, H. (1992). "Health risk changes with a low-cost individualized health promotion program: Effects at up to 30 months." *American Journal of Health Promotion* 6, 364-371.

34. Nieman, D.C. (2003). *Exercise Testing and Prescription a Health Related Approach.* (pp. 1-22). New York, NY: McGraw-Hill Higher Education.

35. Yen, L., Edington, D.W., & Whitting, P. (1991). "Association between health risk appraisal scores and employees medical claims costs in a manufacturing company." *American Journal of Health Promotion* 6, 46-54.

36. Jeffery, R. (1993). "Effects of worksite health promotion on Illinois-related absenteeism." *Journal of Occupational Medicine* 35, 1142-1146.

37. Knight, K. (1994). "An evaluation of Duke University's Live for Life health promotion program on changes in worker absenteeism." *Journal of Occupational Medicine* 36, 533-534.

38. Aldana, S.G. (2001). "Health Promotion Programs, Modifiable Health Risks, and Employee Absenteeism." *Journal of Occupational and Environmental Medicine* 43(1) 36-46.

39. Leutzinger, J.A., Ozminkowski, R.J., Dunn, R.L., Goetzel, R.Z., Richling, D.E., Stewart, M., Whitmer R.W. "Projecting Future Medical Care Costs Using Four Different Scenarios of Lifestyle Risk Rates." *American Journal of Health Promotion* 15(1) 35-44.

CHAPTER SEVEN

COMPREHENSIVE REVIEW OF HEALTH PROMOTION PROGRAMS

This chapter provides a comprehensive review of selected health promotion programs from across the country. During the course of this chapter, numerous companies and organizations will be introduced. National and international companies, public as well as private, large, and small, community based, student based, and corporate based programs have been included. Extensive research, data, and statistical analyses on program efficacy, physiological efficacy, and return on investment (ROI) studies are presented.

From exercise facilities to free childcare, these are just some of the promotional programs in place to encourage the overall well-being of employees. When a company adopts a health promotion or wellness program they may be doing it for a multitude of reasons: (1) to reduce the costs of health care, (2) to join an already booming trend among high profile companies, (3) to improve employee morale, productivity, and reduce absenteeism, and/or (4) to improve employee health. Irregardless of the reason, this ever growing trend seems to be catching on. Healthy employees translate into productive employees that can lead to increased productivity and increased profit margin for employers. To employers it may seem minor, but they are providing a service that benefits their employees in more ways than one. First, they are showing that they care about their employees. When workers can see that the management is concerned with personal issues and well being, they tend to give more effort to the job they are performing. A little time on behalf of the senior staff can mean great improvements to employee morale and confidence.

Management's show of concern for the employees physical health can lead to many improvements in the workers overall attitude. When the workers physical health improves, they feel better and that can be portrayed in many different capacities. By helping an employee with their physical health, the person may become less stressful about a situation, gain self-confidence and improve self-esteem. This increased self-confidence and self-esteem may lead to better work production from that particular employee. Multiply this effect by the number of employees within a business and great dividends can accrue.

The benefits may be accrued in a fitness facility or by educating the employees' on how to mange stress. Many individuals are uninformed as to what they should and should not do when it comes to their health. Studies have demonstrated that once educated about their health, people can make significant improvements. By exercising in a fitness facility, a person can gain psychologically as well as physiologically. Physical exercise is a great way to reduce stress and anxiety. If education is something that a company chooses to do then simple seminars at lunchtime have shown effectiveness. Seminars can be on time management, exercise, stress management, cholesterol, blood pressure, or healthy eating habits. Integral program components of a multitude of health promotion, fitness and wellness programs follow. Program mission and vision statements, leadership and staff information, and statistical data on return on investment studies are included.

Components of each program are categorized and defined

according to the three levels of prevention: primary, secondary, and tertiary. Primary prevention intervention strategies include programs, and services that *prevent the clinical manifestation* of a disease or a condition. Within primary prevention, two strategies are employed. The first involves modifying the environment. Examples of this include eliminating unhealthy snacks from vending machines, and implementing "no smoking" policies. The goal of this intervention strategy is to deliberately manipulate the environment so that the person has no choice, but to adopt a healthier lifestyle. Unhealthy choices are eliminated from the environment. This is the most successful approach to creating healthy environments. The second venue within primary prevention is to modify the individual, through encouragement, increased awareness, and education. This approach is less successful because it requires volition and assumes the person will make the healthier choice when given proper information. It is the intervention strategy most often employed in health promotion programming.

The second level of prevention strategies is called secondary prevention. Secondary prevention aims at *early detection*, and is employed when a disease or a condition cannot be prevented. Examples of secondary prevention include cancer screenings, blood pressure screenings, and cholesterol screenings.

The third level of prevention strategies is called tertiary prevention, and involves *maximizing functional capacity* in the presence of a disease or a condition. Examples of this are cardiac rehabilitation programs, physical therapy, and cancer support groups.

Each level of prevention is important, and all are necessary for complete and comprehensive health promotion programming. The programs reviewed in this chapter are listed alphabetically.

AUGSBURG COLLEGE FACULTY AND STAFF FITNESS AND WELLNESS PROGRAM

Augsburg College, a higher education institution with 3,000 students, is located in Minneapolis, Minnesota. They have developed and implemented a faculty and staff fitness and wellness Program that is designed to make it easier and more convenient for the employees to exercise on campus.

Augsburg College is concerned about the well being of its personnel. Many opportunities are available to the faculty and staff as a member of Augsburg College. The Center for Counseling and Health Promotion offers a counseling staff available to the faculty and staff for consultations and for referrals regarding personal issues. Throughout the year, the staff of the Center for Counseling and Health Promotion offers many campus health events such as guest lectures and health fairs.

The fitness and wellness programs include a multitude of services such as: incentive and reward programs, and fitness programs. The facility consists of a pool, two tennis courts, ice arena, racquetball court, a fitness facility, and athletic fields. Activities can be designed specifically to meet the needs of the Augsburg faculty and staff, who are encouraged to participate.

The unique feature of this program is that members of the college's faculty and staff are eligible to earn points towards prizes for exercising. Employees must report their workout days and dates each week (exercise frequency) and include name, department, telephone extension, type of activity, and exercise duration. Employees can also receive points for exercising at home. When an employee reaches 150 points the employees name is placed into a random drawing whereby the winner receives $100.00 off their health insurance premium. This represents a significant paradigm shift, as the employer is contributing to and financially rewarding improved employee health, as opposed to the traditional model of simply paying for treatment. It represents a valid prevention program.

AETNA

Aetna is one of the nations leading providers of health care, dental, pharmacy, group life, disability, and long-term care products, and serves over 37 million clients. With headquarters in

Connecticut, Aetna provides five high quality fitness centers for its employees, and for those who choose not to participate in these centers, the company offers discount memberships to health clubs in conjunction with Global Fit.

Through extensive research and data analysis, Aetna has concluded that the employees who make use of these fitness centers cost them $282 less per year than do those employees who do not exercise. Other contributing factors to healthier, and money saving employees is the number of services Aetna has to offer its employees and their families. Among these are screenings for early detection of common diseases and cancers (secondary prevention), and child vaccinations to guard against diseases (primary prevention).

Aetna is also concerned with improving the quality of their employees' lives. The company offers a smoking cessation program to educate the employees about health and behavior risks, and has established a smoke-free environment throughout the company (primary prevention). Smoking cessation is one of the biggest steps people can take to improve their health. Realizing this, Aetna offers the Healthy Breathing Program. This program is an eight to twelve week smoking cessation program that uses nicotine replacement therapy and a personal quit plan to help smokers break their addiction to cigarettes.

Aetna provides notable and highly regarded health promotion and disease prevention services for women. The Association for Female Executives has rewarded these outstanding programs and services by recognizing Aetna as a "Top 30 Company for Women Executives" for the 5th straight year.

Programs and services for women include a breast cancer case management program, annual screenings for cervical, breast, and colorectal cancers, direct access for obstetrical or gynecological care, and a moms-to-babies maternity management program. Aetna also offers education for women who are considering pregnancy but have a health risk such as diabetes, programs for women who may want to inquire about infertility treatment, and services for women who may have questions about menopause.

Aetna's health promotion program contains many components and services for its employees. Among these components are means for early recognition and detection (secondary prevention). Beginning at age 40, female members receive educational information about menopause. This includes a take-at-home osteoporosis self-evaluation. In terms of mammography, beginning annually at age 40, each female member receives information, which stresses the importance of mammography, breast self-examinations, and annual gynecologic exams. This information may also include a referral to a participating mammography center. Information on colorectal cancer is distributed to employees. A kit to test for blood in the stool as a possible early sign of cancer is also sent with instructions on how to complete the test. Following the completion of the test, the employee's physician receives the results and a letter is sent to the employee stating the results are available through their primary care physician's office. Also, annually, starting at 18 years of age, female members are sent information stressing the importance of annual gynecological exams and a recommendation to schedule one. In addition, women who have not had a pap smear in two and two and a half years are sent a reminder to schedule and exam as soon as possible.

Aetna also offers a Moms-to-Babies Maternity Management Program, which helps members give their babies a healthy start with educational materials and services. This program includes, assistance in accessing prenatal care benefits, case management by a registered nurse who will review the program's features and answer any questions. Also, a smoke-free Moms-to-be program is designed specifically for pregnant women, and a comprehensive pregnancy handbook which includes detailed information on prenatal care, labor, and delivery, newborn care, nursing and feeding, postpartum depression, and other pregnancy-related health issues.

Aetna cares about their employee's children as well. To promote good health through primary prevention, Aetna sends out a birthday card reminder containing a recommended immunization schedule.

Aetna developed the Poison Prevention Program to provide eligible employees with information on how to protect themselves and their families against accidental poisoning, and how best to respond to the event of a poisoning emergency. Member families with children five years and younger are sent an educational packet. The packet includes a home safety guide that can help them prevent accidental poisoning and tells them what to do in case of an emergency (primary prevention).

Nutrition is also important, and Aetna's Healthy Eating booklet outlines the benefits of a healthy diet and provides information on how to get started. It focuses on helping employees understand and use the Food Guide Pyramid, read the "Nutrition Facts" label on foods, lower the amount of fat intake, and become more physically active (primary prevention).

Regular activity and overall fitness can help an employee achieve good physical health. It can also offer psychological and emotional benefits, help manage and control weight, promote psychological well being, and can reduce stress and help an employee look and feel their best. Aetna provides discounts on membership rates, offers monthly memberships with no long term contracts, allows monthly billing of fitness dues to the employees checking or savings account, gives free guest passes, and offers discounts on certain home exercise equipment in order to promote the idea of regular physical activity (primary prevention).

Finally, the last three programs to be reviewed are aimed at helping employees and their physicians better manage chronic disease (tertiary prevention). The first is Aetna's Asthma Management Program, which integrates comprehensive asthma education and instruction in the use of asthma management equipment designed for home use. The next is the Diabetes Management Program, which combines employee education with blood glucose self-monitoring to help achieve better blood glucose control and reduce the probability for diabetic complications to occur. The final program is the Low Back Pain Disease Management Program, which provides access to educational materials to help prevent recurrent low back pain.

The community is important to Aetna. In the southeast region of the country, Aetna donated $125,000, of which $95,000 will be directed to health programs for the Community Grants Program. Since 1997, Aetna has supplied over $8 million to women's cardiovascular health services. Aetna intends that this money will help raise health awareness, education, and prevention initiatives aimed at decreasing the incidence of cardiovascular disease.

Aetna has twice been awarded the C. Everett Koop National Health Award demonstrating that these programs are of high quality, comprehensive, and serve as excellent resources and benefits for the employees of Aetna.

BRIGHAM YOUNG UNIVERSITY

A Mormon university with 30,000 students, Brigham Young University (BYU) is located in Provo, Utah. The Wellness Program at BYU has been established since 1998. The multidimensional program contains physical, social, spiritual, emotional, financial, and intellectual components including: physical fitness activities, education, clinics/screenings, programs, a schedule of events, and a newsletter. The program mission statement is: "An ongoing program encourages university personnel and their families to strengthen their health and well being through educational opportunities, clinics, fun wellness activities, self-improvement, and 'Y Be Fit'".

The 'Y Be Fit' program is the cornerstone of the wellness initiative. There are three components included in this program coordinated by faculty and students. First, pre-program assessments determine the person's present health status. Second, an education and activity prescription for the individual follows. Finally, there is follow-up counseling to ensure healthy and positive outcomes. There are also personnel, facilities, and a host of websites to use as resources.

The schedule of events includes different recreational tournaments. There are also various fitness challenges, along with several fun-run activities. Recognizing the importance of social needs, the goal is to define fitness as a social event. As part of the education program, articles containing several health issues are posted. Health fairs, workshops, and seminars are listed along with dates, times and locations. This provides an excellent opportunity for people to learn about different issues. There is a question and answer board open for anyone to use as a resource to learn. A newsletter called *Well News* is comprised of monthly articles to update those interested in current research.

Numerous screenings are offered as well as risk stratification programs for those who do not pass the initial screenings. Included in the assessment are screenings of: blood pressure, bone density, breast cancer, cholesterol, fitness, glucose analysis, influenza vaccination, nutrition profile, and prostate cancer. All are very important and each is available to the university staff and their families.

CATERPILLAR

With its corporate headquarters located in Peoria, Illinois, Caterpillar is the words largest manufacturer of construction and mining equipment, diesel and natural gas engines, and industrial gas turbines. With annual sales of $9.70 billion, Caterpillar has 72,000 employees. Developed over a three-year period, and introduced in 1997, the employee based wellness program is called the Healthy Balance. The program foundation, which was enhanced and modified by Caterpillar, is called HealthTrac®. The funding for this program is from the executive office of the Caterpillar Company.

There are 142 United States of America and International sites for the Healthy Balance program. The staff consists of highly qualified professionals, including seven full-time staff in the medical department ranging from health promotion manager to data analysis and communicators. Part-time staff consists primarily of nurses, physicians, and health educators. The nurses specialize in diabetes and cardiac care. The physicians specialize in infectious disease, occupational health, and public health. There are also ninety-one additional part time employees at the 142 sites.

PROGRAM DESIGN

The Healthy Balance Program incorporates best practice features. In order to design a high quality program, the health promotion literature was reviewed and 21 companies with outstanding health promotion programs were benchmarked. The HealthTrac® Program, significantly modified and enhanced by Caterpillar, is the program's foundation.

One key ingredient to Healthy Balance is strong incentives. A second feature is top down management "buy-in" and involvement. The third component is that an individuals' spouse is permitted to join the program. This is advantageous for increasing social support, as the couple can participate together. The final feature is a process involving continuous evaluation to constantly improve services and programs for the employees.

The first goal for Healthy Balance is to motivate positive behavioral change. The second goal is to reduce health risks, and improve long-term health status. The third goal of the program is to promote self-efficiency, and informed decision making. The fourth goal is to reduce healthcare costs. The fifth and final goal of Healthy Balance is to achieve exceptional participation via strong incentives.

PROGRAM COMPONENTS

- Low-cost confidential health assessments
- Focus on modifiable risks and increasing self-efficacy
- Personalized health education messages
- Stratification into low and high risk categories and periodic assessments based on risk
- Individualized interventions, targeted to health risks and readiness-to-change
- Intensive high risk and chronic condition interventions, including disease management phone counseling
- Serial tracking and ongoing monitoring and adjustment of interventions

- Coordination with related interventions (on-site classes, referral to community programs, etc.)
- Self-care book and quarterly newsletters to all eligible employees
- Toll-free health information line and audio library
- Intranet website regularly updated, linked to sites providing scientifically validated information
- Ongoing evaluation using integrated data warehouse (claims, absenteeism, etc.) and communication of summary results to the employees

TARGET POPULATION

All U.S. – based non-union employees (49% of workforce) and spouses (N=41,500+).
To be added: retirees, union workers (pending contract changes).

CATERPILLAR HEALTHY BALANCE OUTCOMES

As reported by Caterpillar, and based upon analysis of the population's baseline health risks, and the success of the Healthy Balance Program to date, it is anticipated that the long-term savings will be more than $700 million by 2015. The evaluation of participation, retention, self-reported risk and use of healthcare services, satisfaction, and baseline versus current claims expenditures reveals that the program has achieved outstanding results:

- High Participation: 96% of eligible employees, and 74% of eligible spouses
- Reduction in risk factors: The health risk score, as determined by HealthTrac®, decreased 6% for the low risk population (N=22,114). For the population (N= 2,321) completing the entire high-risk program (a series of five health assessments and health education interventions), health risk declined by 14%. Decrease

in aggregate risk represents improvement in the major risk factors including physical activity, cigarette smoking, stress, fat, and fiber consumption, etc.

- Savings: Participants who completed the high risk program reduced their frequency of doctor office visits by 17% and hospital days by 28%, resulting in a 23% decrease in direct costs, validated by claims data.
- Reduction in claims costs. Between 1997 and 1999, average claims for non-eligible employees (N=13,291) increased at a much higher rate (40% faster) than did those for participants (N=12,932).
- Cost savings for those with heart disease. Heart disease is Caterpillar's highest contributor to healthcare costs. In a small case/control study (age/gender matched) of employees who had heart disease prior to the start of the program, participants who completed more than one health assessment (N=8) had lower medical claims costs than did non-participants (N=50). Over the 3-year study period, average per person claims costs were $16,121. lower for participants than non-participants.
- Smoking cessation. 1,144 participants quit smoking cigarettes.
- Reduction in body mass index (BMI). Overweight is regarded as Caterpillar's #1 preventable health risk. At the start of the program, more than 60% of eligible employees had a BMI greater than 25. Since the implementation of the program, more than 4,700 of this group have attained a lower BMI.
- External recognition. The program won the Dr. Solovy Community Health Award, given by a panel of business leaders and University of Illinois professors.
- Internal review/Continuous Quality Improvement processes. Continuous improvement is achieved by ongoing evaluation and dissemination of program results. A satisfaction survey is being conducted.

COORS BREWING COMPANY

More than twenty years ago, in 1981, chairman Bill Coors believing that "wellness and health care cost management go together", initiated a wellness program at Coors Brewing Company in Golden Colorado. Since its inception, Coors has received National Recognition while being honored with awards such as: The C. Everett Koop National Health Award in 1992 &1995, The *Human Resource Executive* magazine's benchmark company in 1992, and *Club Industry* magazine's Titan of Corporate Fitness in 1992.

The Coors wellness program addresses lifestyle issues and focuses on primary, secondary, and tertiary levels of prevention. The program includes a multitude of services and programs including health risk appraisals, health screenings, nutrition education and counseling, aerobic exercise classes and exercise equipment, orthopedic conditioning and rehabilitation as well as cardiac rehabilitation, and physical therapy.

Overall, Coors wellness program has had a very high rate of return. According to internal research, for every $1 spent on its corporate wellness program there is a return of $6.20. The cardiac rehabilitation program has reported a significant impact on this high rate of return. Over six years the cardiac rehabilitation program saved the company $1,390,661. The program requires employees and their dependents to participate in the program if they have experienced a cardiac event.

An initiative that makes Coors' special is their Employment Opportunity Training Program, called "The Golden Door". This program teaches people who are educationally, economically, and socially disadvantaged how to become reliable, and productive employees. Included in this training are mandatory GED certifications for those without a diploma. The rate of success for this program is quite remarkable. Since 1977 about 75% of the trainees who entered the program have taken regular production and office jobs throughout Coors. About 50% of these employees have remained with the company.

CHEVRON

Another business that was a recipient of the C. Everett Koop National Health Award is the Chevron Corporation. With its headquarters located in San Ramon, California, Chevron is one of the largest refiners and marketers of petroleum products in the United States. The goal of Chevron's program, called Healthy Quest, is to provide services that promote a healthy and productive workplace. An integrated approach between an interdisciplinary staff of health professionals insures that employees' mental and physical needs are addressed. Comprehensive fitness centers are available for the employees, and the transtheoretical model of behavior change is incorporated. The average age of the employees is forty-seven and the average years of service is eighteen. Approximately sixty percent of the people are traditionally classified as "blue collar", which includes employees in the refineries to the chemical plants. The company has employees throughout the United States of America but mostly concentrated in the Gulf Coast and California. The participation rate for Chevron employees is approximately seventy percent.

The goals for Healthy Quest are to reduce health risk (primary and secondary prevention). The second goal is to reduce absenteeism from work. The third goal is to reduce on-site and off-site injuries. The final goal is to reduce costs associated with health care.

CIGNA CORPORATION - WORKING WELL LIVING WELL

CIGNA has consolidated assets of $95.1 billion and is a huge provider of health care, insurance, and financial services. With its headquarters in Philadelphia, Working Well is CIGNA Corporation's initiative to keep its 33,000 U.S. employees healthy, and at work. The program has an annual budget of $3.5 million, and has been implemented at all of its 365 domestic offices. Working Well has a broad range of programs for all employees and utilizes local site coordinators to maintain a human interface with employees. Recognized by *Working Mothers Magazine* as one of the top 100 companies for working mothers for the 10th consecutive year, the company is known for family friendly programs, and its programs place special emphasis on issues of concern to women who make up 80% of CIGNA's population.

KEY PROGRAMS INCLUDE:

Working Well Moms - CIGNA's lactation program was the subject of a study conducted by the ULCA Center for Healthier Children, Families and Communities. Results of the study revealed that the program is exceeding its defined goals as listed below:

- Breast feeding initiation and duration rates exceed the Healthy People 2010 Objectives
- Breast feeding duration rates for participants are 72 percent at 6 months, significantly higher than control groups and US data
- Decreased pharmacy costs: 62 percent fewer prescriptions for breast-fed children
- Decreased medical cost: the program saves the company $240,000 in healthcare expenses
- Reduced absenteeism: program participants have 74 fewer absences/100 mothers, a savings of $60,000 in lost time annually
- Removed socioeconomic disparities in participants so that job grade and education were not predicators of breastfeeding at six and 12 months

Triumph - a voluntary personalized lifestyle modification program, CIGNA's Triumph program was the subject of an internal study comprised of pre and post-test evaluation to measure changes in health risk resulting from the program. Results of the study (listed below) revealed that the program is effective in reaching the company's highest risk short-term disability population.

- 86 percent met personalized health goals
- Significant reduction in health risks in four of the five greatest risks
- Improvement in health inventory scores. Increases observed in both the Mental Component Summary (pre-intervention score was 40 and the post-intervention score was 45); and Physical Component Summary (pre-intervention score of 41 to post score of 44).
- Healthcare costs savings of $162. per program participant

Osteoporosis Screening - CIGNA expanded its osteoporosis-screening program this year, and 1,124 employees participated. An internal evaluation was based on three data sources: demographic and risk factor data obtained at the time of the screening, specific T scores, and a six month post screening survey. Results suggest that the program met and/or exceeded the defined goals, including:

- 170 employees had osteopenia; 14 percent with osteoporosis were initially categorized after taking a risk assessment
- 62 percent with abnormal results discussed them with their primary care physician; 42 percent had pDEXA scans and 38 percent started medication
- 92 percent initiated at least 1 behavior change with an average of 3.5
- 75 percent talked to daughters and mothers about reducing osteoporosis risk

Flu Shots - This national program reached 12,500 CIGNA employees in 1999. The program was evaluated internally with a survey of 2,471 employees at nine CIGNA worksites. Respondents who qualified for flu shots and their attendance data were evaluated for the 1999-2000 flu season. The results (listed below) demonstrated that the program resulted in a positive return on investment in the employee population.

- 29 percent less absenteeism vs. employees not getting a flu shot (122 workdays absent versus 157 days absent per 100 employees)
- 54 percent did not miss work due to flu or upper respiratory illness
- Savings of $33 per employee was realized in lost time
- Total program cost was $141,250. Overall return on investment was 3:1 ($412,500 saved vs. $141,500 cost)

DAIMLER CHRYSLER/UAW NATIONAL WELLNESS PROGRAM

Daimler Chrysler Corporation is a leading international automotive and transportation company with over 95,000 employees throughout the United States, and 365,600 world-wide. With revenues of $158 billion, Daimler Chrysler has its headquarters in Auburn Hills, Michigan.

The Daimler Chrysler/UAW National Wellness Program, which began in 1985, is a negotiated benefit between Daimler Chrysler Corporation and the International Union of Auto Workers, the UAW. Several national health and fitness service providers are contracted health and fitness partners (over 100FTEs) to administer the Program. The Daimler Chrysler Human Resources Department provides operating funds for the Program and with the UAW, provides administrative oversight.

The program provides high quality, cost-effective wellness activities that empower employees to improve their health and become wise health care consumers while containing health care costs. Specific Program objectives for 2000 include:

- Screen 37 percent of population to assess risks and interests

- Increase percent of employees who have fewer than 3 health risks
- Increase participation in the *Next Steps TM* Program (phone-based lifestyle intervention targeted to high-risk individuals) by 1% at each site
- Decrease percentage of smokers by 6%

Employees voluntarily participate. Targeted education programs, based on identified health risks and interests, provide an opportunity for individual health improvements. Interventions tailored to individual sites customize the program for each population while maintaining the objectives and quality standards required of all sites.

Focused education programs support employees throughout the process of lifestyle change. The transtheoretical model of behavior change is used for tailoring programs such as smoking cessation, weight management, cholesterol management and fitness activities. Program formats may include one-time workshops, multi-session classes, individual counseling, or self-directed modules. Maintenance strategies include ongoing awareness, interactive campaigns, group support, incentive opportunities, follow-up, and cultural support with on-site services (e.g., fitness facilities, cafeteria/vending programs, and walking routes).

According to research studies, if a high-risk employee were to complete at least one Health Risk Assessment and participate in physical activity or a wellness activity each year, they would be capable of saving Daimler Chrysler $200.35 per year in health care costs. This amount multiplied by the number of employees that actually participate and follow through with this program is a significant amount of money for a company to save. Not only has the company saved in dollar amounts, it has also helped people in making healthy lifestyle and positive behavioral changes. More people are eating healthy, quitting smoking, and more have a fewer number of risk factors. This is attributed to their participation in this program.

The program prides itself in achieving high standards in health promotion. Some of the awards the program has received include:

- Well Workplace Gold Awards (Wellness Council of America, 23 in 1998, 8 in 1999)
- Governor's Council on Physical Fitness (Gold Awards, 1997)
- Healthiest Corporate Cafeteria (Physicians Committee for Research and Medicine, 1997)

IMPACT OF STAYWELL PROGRAMS ON CHRYSLER HEALTH CARE COSTS, 1999

Researchers of the University of Rochester used a multivariate regression analysis to estimate the effects of the Wellness Program on 1997 healthcare cost. Pertinent details include:

- The study included 38,318 employees from 10 Chrysler sites enrolled in either traditional indemnity insurance or PPO insurance between 1992 and 1997 and who completed at least one Health Risk Assessment (HRA)
- To detect and control for possible selection effects, program effects were split into components: the impact on health care costs on each risk factor and the effect of each program on the probability of developing a risk factor

The results demonstrated that health risk assessment (HRA) completion is associated with significant and substantial cost reductions. Employees who complete one, two or three HRAs on average had lower 1997 health care costs of $112.89, $134.22, and $152.29 respectively. Regarding the association of health care costs and the presence of health risks, and consistent with other published research, most of the health risks were shown to increase health care costs, and an increase in the number of risk factors increased health care costs.

HEALTH RISKS AND THEIR IMPACT ON MEDICAL COSTS

A study representing 6,000 life-years of UAW/Chrysler employees over a three-year period confirmed risk-cost linkages. The results demonstrated that individuals with the following health risks had higher claims costs as compared to those at low-risk:

- Smokers, 31% higher
- Unhealthy eating habits, 41% higher
- Stress, 42% higher
- Mental health risks, 13% higher
- Employees outside the healthy weight range, 143% higher hospital inpatient utilization

MANAGEMENT SUMMARY DATA

Data based on 18,638 employees who completed an HRA in 1999 and at least one other HRA in the past. The average time between initiation and completion was 3.4 years. The following changes in risk were evident:

- Eating habits improved 16%
- Smoking risk decreased 15%
- Participants with six or more risks decreased 6%
- Participants with fewer than three risks improved 5%. Based on the changes in the health risks of repeat participants, the program estimates annual savings of $5,908,600.

HEALTH ACTIVITY CENTER PHYSICAL PERFORMANCE DATA

Data from general fitness assessments at the Health Activity Center provide evidence of measurable improvements in cardiovascular conditioning and in blood pressure.

PARTICIPANT SATISFACTION

Satisfaction surveys are conducted upon completion of programs (courses, screenings, and work-shops) on an ongoing basis. Satisfaction rates exceeded 95% in both 1998 and 1999.

DOW CHEMICAL COMPANY

Headquartered in Chicago, Dow chemical company is the fifth largest chemical company in the world with 39,000 employees and $20 billion in sales. The American College of Occupational and Environmental Medicine (ACOEM) named the Dow Chemical Company, one of the three national winners in its 2000 ACOEM Corporate Health Achievement Awards. Included among the many positive outcomes of Dow's health and safety initiatives that qualified them to earn this honor was the steady reduction in reportable incidents. The reportable incident rates dropped from 2.07 in 1995 to 1.60 in 1996, 1.66 in 1997, 1.27 in 1998, and a further reduction in 1999. Within three years there was also a reported 90% drop in on-the-job strains and sprains. Supplementing these achievements is data demonstrating that up to 95% of employees in many locations participate in the company's health assessment program. The company also publicizes and uses data obtained through systematic epidemiological and toxicological research in its personal and environmental protection programs in order to benefit employees, communities, and the industry. Dow has conducted more than 100 studies in the past twenty years, examining such areas as cancer incidence and chemical related mortality as well as the cost effectiveness of its health programs and their impact on employee wellness. Positive results from these studies have helped to secure ongoing senior management support for their health promotion program.

The ACOEM singled out the following components of Dow Chemical's benefits program as exemplary model practices. The company's extensive use of web-based intranet for global education, training, publication of guidelines and standards, and data collection. Dow's intranet provides an exceptional and comprehensive resource for all employees by offering them immediate, continuous access to a wide range of information. The information includes health education and wellness materials on a myriad of topics, the written standard for Dow's employee health assessment program. The information also includes (and is updated by a global team of health professionals) information on the current regulations and medical research, and provides search capabilities for the extensive toxicology database on chemicals used at Dow. Training programs on such topics as the correct use of various chemicals (including asbestos, benzene, and butadiene), avoiding general workplace hazards (such as ergonomic injuries, heat stress, and hearing loss), and important health-related issues (like behavior-based safety practices) are incorporated. Health professionals routinely visit different Dow plants and work sites to contribute their knowledge and observations about employee health and safety as a way to help eliminate risks and accidents. These visits are prompted by various circumstances, including, the need to review job conditions, procedure changes that might impact health-related monitoring, or protective equipment needs, or health-related questions from plant management or employees.

DUKE UNIVERSITY EXECUTIVE HEALTH PROGRAM

Duke University is located in Durham, North Carolina and has an enrollment of 11,000 students. Consistent with its human resources goal, and in order to promote a work culture and environment that supports healthy and safe behavior and lifestyles, three programs, The Duke Diet and Fitness Center, Duke Executive Health Program, and Duke Health and Fitness Center are coordinated. All three programs have consistent philosophies of health and wellness. They help create a customized, practical, and sustainable lifestyle plan for each person.

The programs, collectively named, "Live for Life", are open to all employees. Services include: health screenings, fitness and injury prevention programs, and programs in stress management, nutrition, and weight loss. Smoking cessation programs as well as blood pressure and cholesterol screenings are included. "Pathways to Change", a personal counseling service is provided to assist with behavioral change. A unique feature of the program is that the participants can record their lifestyle activity record on the web site and in doing so, earn live for life dollars that can be used to purchase items in the live for life store.

Duke Executive Health Program is located in the Duke Center that sits on a beautiful 26-acre wooded area. The center is adjacent to Duke University, and Duke University Medical Center. Duke University Medical Center developed a web site called Activhealth that offers a more extensive online health assessment, the latest information on topics and research in preventive health and personal health development.

Duke Executive Health Programs mission is to help people achieve optimal health and quality of life through prevention, treatment, education, and research. Employees with special healthcare needs can spend two days at the Duke Executive Program and concentrate on special health concerns. Each participant leaves knowing their health status, and is provided with a program that is individually designed to improve their lifestyle and to reduce their risk factors. Employees can receive additional testing. These assessments include: prostate-specific antigen (PSA), thyroid profile, sexually transmitted disease & HIV screening, ophthalmic examination, glaucoma test, immunizations for general health and international travel, pulmonary capacity assessment, hearing acuity test, and consultations with Duke specialty physicians. The Duke Executive Health Programs fit into the employee's busy schedule and makes a difference in their health status.

The staff at the Duke Center for Living will work to develop a customized and individualized health plan. Initially, participants are given a comprehensive physiological exam and a health risk assessment that focuses on the major issues of stress, fitness, and nutrition. This is used to develop an individual wellness plan.

As part of Duke University Health System, employees have access to the centers of excellence, including the Duke

Comprehensive Cancer Center, Duke Heart Center, Duke University Eye Center, the Arthritis Center, Women's Services and the Aesthetic Center, and other medical resources.

DUPONT

The DuPont Chemical Company has 79,000 employees, and $24 billion in revenue. Initially an explosives manufacturer (gunpowder) in the 1800's, DuPont has grown into a huge industrial and service corporation, and manufacturers paints, plastics, rayon, nylon, cellophane, freon, Kevlar, Teflon, and Stainmaster carpet.

DuPont has had an employee health promotion program since 1984. Within the first fifteen years, eighty-nine thousand people have had the opportunity to participate in this program. The seven health areas the program focuses on are: stress management, smoking cessation, weight and lipid control, fitness, dental care, and a healthy back. Based on a confidential and individual health assessment, employees attend wellness activities and sessions that are educational.

The costs and benefits are weighed very carefully. Published literature discusses the associated benefits of good health and fitness. Physical activity can help with weight management, muscular strength, and cardiovascular endurance. Self-concept and a positive attitude are usually gained through improvement of overall health. This can lead to good work relationships, and increased productivity. Absenteeism and employee turnover rates have decreased, along with health care costs. Insurance premiums decreased with the implementation of the employee health and wellness program. A positive return on investment was also reported. In Delaware, $1.2 million was invested in The DuPont Company's Health and Wellness Program, with estimated savings of $5 for every $1 invested.

Direct communication with the employees is considered as an important venue to provide information about the program. "Eye catching" information concerning objectives, addressing attitudes and concerns, organizations, and the means to participate in the program are defined. Surveys and seminars encourage employee participation, and promote a feeling of importance.

A needs assessment is utilized and becomes the cornerstone to the development of an evaluation. The evaluation also ensures the success of the program in all areas. Different types of evaluations are used, including outcome evaluation, and impact evaluation. Data management and statistical analysis are also incorporated into the evaluation.

There are a number of challenges associated with health promotion programming, including fostering participation and motivating the employees to fully participate. High quality physical examinations must be provided to ensure proper care of the employees throughout the program. The DuPont Company will continue the program due to the ongoing success both the employees and the company has achieved.

FANNIE MAE

Fannie Mae is the nation's largest home lender, and was created by the U.S. government in 1938 to help the housing industry after the great depression. In 1968, it became a private shareholder owned company, and today, with its 4,700 employees, Fannie Mae has helped 43 million families secure financing for homes.

The Fannie Mae Partnership for Healthy Living is the designated name of Fannie Mae's health promotion and wellness program. With possibly one of the most comprehensive screening protocols, this program is designed to reduce absenteeism, improve overall health, control medical costs, and improve productivity in the work place. Fannie Mae offers this program to all employees and their spouses or domestic partners. There are four components in this program: screening, planning, health promotion, and evaluation. In order to properly design a program to fit the needs of the individual, the screening process in very thorough. Components include:

- Health Assessment Questionnaires
- Health Interest Surveys
- Blood Pressure
- Height/Weight
- Laboratory Testing
- Body Composition
- Bone Mineral Density
- Lung Function
- Mammography
- Influenza Vaccines
- Glaucoma
- Vision
- Fitness Testing
- Tuberculosis
- Personal Wellness Profile (PWP)

Program Managers then develop an implementation plan based on the results of the screening and survey, the previous year's evaluation, and resource availability. The program is customized to meet the distinct needs of each regional office while conforming to general protocol.

The health promotion phase includes group feedback sessions on the personal wellness program (PWP), on-site behavioral modification programs (aerobics, yoga, smoking cessation, weight management), health assessments, lunchtime seminars, walking programs, and a high-risk intervention program. Participation incentives support each health promotion event, including a Healthy Living day off for employees who participate in a health assessment and group feedback session.

The managers of the Partnership for Healthy Living Program evaluate the program based on participation, aggregate health data, health trends, high-risk outcomes, cost-benefit studies, anecdotal reports and surveys from employees. New screening and health promotion practices are reviewed and considered for inclusion.

Fannie Mae has a 60-70% participation rate and a repeat

participation rate of 80%. 90% of the employees who complete the Health Assessment attend a group feedback session, where their results are disseminated and discussed. The total number of high-risk employees has declined and most of those who started as non-high risk remained in that risk stratification. Satisfaction surveys revealed that 80% of Fannie Mae's program participants were satisfied with the program.

This program has received national accolades as Working Woman chose it as the best woman's health promotion program in 1996. More recently, in 2003, the National Association for Female Executives named it a "Top 30" company for executive women (ranked 5th), and Fortune Magazine rated it a "100 Best" companies to work for.

FITNESS USA

Since 1958, Fitness USA Supercenters have been providing corporate health promotion and fitness services to a variety of companies. With offices in Michigan, Indiana, and California, each USA Supercenter provides a wide variety of state of the art fitness equipment and a whirlpool relaxation area. They also offer various forms of high and low step and water aerobics, at no additional cost. They work to demonstrate to the employees the benefits of being physically fit. They offer special corporate membership rates, and pledge to provide excellent service for their members.

They provide each member with a properly supervised and individualized fitness program. At every open enrollment, each employee will receive, at no cost, a computerized body fat analysis and report, and a customized fitness program developed by certified personal trainers. Also smoking cessation programs, stress management brochures, and an exclusive nutritional guidance book are available.

Fitness USA offers a trustworthy and reliable pledge of service. They are an expanding company that has been committed to serving its members. Their approach to health education and personal improvement is respected. They give each member the opportunity to meet with a certified personal trainer. The trainers will work with each employee to create an individualized program that suits their goals and needs. They work with the employees to maximize their exercise time. They also teach the employees about healthy eating and proper nutrition. Aerobic dance classes are available and are offered with no additional charge. They are very committed to having employees exercise in their fitness center. They do an excellent job of providing an environment where the employee can feel comfortable and have all their questions and concerns addressed by a qualified personal trainer.

Overall, they provide a dynamic health and fitness program that will introduce, encourage, and educate employees on the importance of leading a healthy lifestyle. Fitness USA claims that there will be immediate benefits after the employees use the fitness programs created for them. Some of those benefits are a decrease in absenteeism, and improved job performance and morale. They believe that fit employees feel better about work and about their job, and that this will translate into increased productivity

HAYWOOD REGIONAL MEDICAL CENTER

Haywood Regional Medical Center, founded in 1927, is located in the Smoky Mountains of Western North Carolina. A public facility, the Health and Fitness Center is available to the general population. The Health Promotion Department developed an employee wellness program called, WellCheck. This represents the incentive based employee wellness program that has been in existence since 1996. The program is available for all part-time and full-time Haywood Regional Medical Center employees.

Haywood Regional Health and Fitness Centers programs goals are to improve and maintain employee's health and well being and to control health care costs. The program consists of the following: health assessments, individual follow-up for high-risk participants, educational classes, and awareness information for employees. Topics such as: nutrition, self-care, safety, mental health, stress management, fitness, alternative health, team based competition, smoking cessation, and family health are available. The Employees of Haywood Medical Center receive a quarterly health newsletter and other corporate wellness services such as: Weight Management Nutritional Services, Out Patient Diabetes Education, and a Health Resource Library. Out Patient Diabetes Education is a physician-referred program that consists of a seven-week education and instruction series. A certified Diabetes Educator provides individual, or group classes, with a support group that meets once a month. They also offer a Living Well Calendar, which is a quarterly publication that lists educational opportunities including: smoking cessation, stress management, and cooking demonstrations. It also includes information about the additional programs and services of Haywood Regional Medical Center.

HEALTHTRAX

Healthtrax is located in Connecticut, and is a health and fitness business that works in conjunction with a number of different companies and hospitals to improve employee health. Founded in 1999, Healthtrax has served over 100,000 people and 375 companies. They provide a network of quality facilities to serve large amounts of employees in different areas. Healthtrax offers an employee wellness program for numerous companies and hospitals including AMICA Insurance, Crowley Chrysler Plymouth, Dairy Mart, Hallmark, Lego Systems, Spalding Sports, Bristol Hospital, and St. Luke's Hospital.

Healthtrax corporate Wellness and Fitness Division has been named the International Health, Racquet, and Sportsclub Association's Employee Wellness Program of the Year, and has been awarded the Michigan Governor's Council on Healthy Workplace Award for six consecutive years (1997-2002). The fact that so many companies are involved with Healthtrax, coupled with the recognition of this award spotlights a highly effective program.

Healthtrax's overall description of their Employee Wellness Program is, "it all adds up to improved morale, increased productivity, a healthier workplace and a solid return on investment." Strategic goals are established for the program. The first goal is a reduction in health care costs. Theoretically, improving the health of an employee will increase his or her own productivity. The accepted axiom, "healthier employees will be absent less" is adopted. Healthtrax wants its clients to achieve a positive return on investment. The program is designed to achieve this goal.

There are a number of services included in a typical Healthtrax program. First, a Health Risk Appraisal is used to establish a baseline for the employees. Healthtrax offers an annual health fair complete with programs and activities. This gives people the opportunity to learn about what is available.

There are personal health screenings offered including cholesterol and body composition. Additionally, a Preventive Case Management program is set up for those employees considered to be "at risk". Self-Help Programs are available on tapes, and booklets, and guides to help people establish their own good health are provided. The value of these programs is allowing people to feel good about themselves by doing it themselves.

A Wellness Newsletter is printed with helpful hints and reminders that guide and inspire employees to better wellness. Home products are available for sale, which can be tested and sampled at the annual wellness fair.

Employee wellness programs include full fitness memberships at all the different network facilities. Employee assistance programs are available, and include thorough physiological assessments, psychological counseling, referrals, and education in any health related area. There are also Wellness Workshops that can educate with guidance and information. This is the core of the employee assistance programs. The quality of these programs has made Healthtrax successful.

JOHNSON & JOHNSON

Since 1979, when Johnson & Johnson created its well-recognized health promotion program, Live for Life, they have been recognized as a leader in health promotion programming. With annual savings of $225. per person and total annual savings of $8.5 million, the program was launched in response to the development of a new employee health strategy. This strategy focused on education and prevention as well as emphasizing both lifestyle modification, and helping employees become better educated as consumers of health care services.

Johnson & Johnson summarizes their strategy with their mission statement: "Health & Wellness provides state-of-the-art Disability Management, Employee Assistance, Occupational Medicine and Wellness services to Johnson & Johnson employees through an integrated, cost-effective approach that meets our customers' and emphasizes prevention and education".

The implementation of this program has resulted in a dramatic reduction in absenteeism within the first two years of implementation. Hospital costs also fell dramatically within the first three years, a reported 34%. The distinguishing characteristic of the program is the $500.00 health care premium discount the employees' receive when they participate in the program. To receive this discount employees must have their blood pressure, cholesterol and body fat measured, as well as complete a questionnaire related to health risks. In 1995 about 96% of J&J's 35,000 employees participated in the program. It is important to recognize that prior to the initiation of premium discount there was only about a 40% participation rate.

Among the many programs and services that Johnson & Johnson provides, their Occupational Injury and Illness Prevention program shines brightly. The professional staff works alongside management and health safety professionals to improve health and safety initiatives in the workplace. The occupational health professionals are primarily responsible for early identification, and treatment of injury and illness of employees. Once an employee is recognized to be at potential risk for workplace hazards they are placed in a health surveillance program. This program provides testing, health evaluations, immunizations, and follow-up examinations.

The Lost Workday Case prevention plan is a combination of preventive initiatives and effective medical case management. This plan works to positively address employee health needs, ensure a safe and proper return to work, and improve morale while minimizing lost productivity.

Johnson & Johnson has an Employee Assistance Program (EAP), that provides professional, and confidential services to help employees and family members resolve personal issues and problems before they affect health, relationships, and job performance. This program is available on a 24-hour, 7 days-a-week basis. Their EAP provides support for a large range of issues including marital/family concerns, financial difficulties, stress, relationship problems, child or elder care concerns, and alcohol/substance abuse. In addition, supervisors are trained in observing behaviors as they relate to job performance, and referring employees for assistance. Johnson & Johnson also encourages and promotes the prevention, identification, and treatment of all mental health and substance abuse issues. In support of a drug-free workplace, Johnson & Johnson has an alcohol and drug policy that is supported by drug testing procedures. Included in this program are alcohol and drug training for their sales force, and EAP supervisory training that provides information on identification of behaviors indicative of substance abuse, and mental health and substance abuse treatment. Coverage is provided through the health care plans offered to the employees.

Additionally, they offer The Return to Wellness Program, which aims to support an employee's return to work, as well as to wellness. The key components of this program are early identification, and providing assistance for their disabilities in a cost-effective way that ensures quality medical care, and a safe and appropriate return to work.

Fall prevention is another program offered. The goal of this program is to prevent falls and injuries, and provide workplace management with the tools to assess the potential for employee injury. The program is designed in phases and incorporates a written program on hazard recognition assistance, engineering consideration, preventative maintenance training, and management techniques.

Specific preventative measures are also taken in Johnson & Johnson's pharmaceutical manufacturing facilities where employees wear personal protective clothing, including respirators to reduce the potential for inhalation or to protect the skin from absorbing the medication.

Another remarkable program offered is the Balancing Work & Family program. Johnson & Johnson recognizes the growing female employee population, and the importance of addressing family dynamics. They offer a very broad and flexible leave policy for family care matters as well as offering adoption benefits, resource and referral programs, and other forms of assistance. On-site child development centers are also available. In New Jersey and Pennsylvania more than 500 children are currently active at these development centers.

Lifeworks is another program which reaches far beyond that of basic health needs. It helps employees to manage their lives outside of work. Counseling and information are provided on topics such as: writing a living will, finding a house-sitter, finding and evaluating child and elder care, improving time-management skills, and developing a home budget.

The final program for review is the Proactive Health Assessments that provide the opportunity for employees to measure their health risks. These screenings provide information on the risks and medical conditions as well as suggest potential solutions. As an example of primary and secondary prevention, counseling, behavior modification, and regular exercise prescriptions are available.

In conclusion, it is well recognized that Johnson & Johnson provides comprehensive health and wellness services. Multiple programs are offered, and services provided through primary, secondary, and tertiary levels of prevention with the goal of maximizing employee health.

KC WELLNESS

Based in Kentucky, KC Wellness, Inc. is a private company offering health, wellness, safety, and injury prevention programs to companies and individuals. Since 1995, organizations have used KC Wellness health promotion strategies to meet their business objectives and gain a competitive advantage. KC Wellness offers individual programs, group programs, and seminars and workshops.

Individual programs give one-on-one support to employees to help them follow through with their health goals. There are several group programs such as health risk assessment, health risk reduction seminar, tobacco cessation, weight management, and a fitness-at-work program. Seminars and workshops that are available are preventative health screenings, a lifestyle and risk management seminar, nutrition education, cholesterol and heart disease, diabetes management, staff wellness, stress management seminar, and a violence-in-the-workplace workshop. KC Wellness also offers Employee Assistance Programs that help bridge the gap between the employees personal concerns and their job performance.

KC Wellness offers a specific substance abuse management program with the objective of creating a drug-free workplace that complies with all federally mandated testing as required by the Department of Transportation and Energy. KC Wellness also offers several group programs such as tobacco cessation, weight management, and health-risk assessment programs. In the tobacco cessation program, the group support can help clients quit smoking or stop chewing tobacco. The program uses behavioral change techniques along with the option of nicotine replacement therapy to achieve a tobacco-free lifestyle. The weight management program promotes a healthy diet for life, focusing on the dietary guidelines for Americans. It also focuses on the importance of physical activity, and coordinates on-site aerobics, stretching, and strength training programs. The health risk assessment (HRA) program provides participants with information about their current health risks, and helps employees learn how to make easy lifestyle changes which will reduce their risk for chronic disease, and increase their quality of life.

The nutrition education provided by KC Wellness includes teaching employees how to apply the national recommendations for a healthy, low fat, high-fiber diet, and how to sort through all the popular fad diets. Employees have the opportunity to also learn the significance of their blood cholesterol levels, and develop strategies to improve the quality of their life as well as to prevent the incidence of heart disease. On-the-job, as well as at home stress-reducing techniques can benefit employees who attend the stress management seminar.

Since type 2 diabetes is a growing public health concern, it would benefit employees greatly to attend the diabetes management program. Issues related to diabetes such as diet and exercise are addressed to educate employees of their risk and strategies and methods to prevent the incidence of diabetes (primary prevention).

It is important to recognize that the leaders and educators of all the programs are certified health education specialists, with teaching experience in diverse settings. Many have over 15 years of experience, and the consultant for the stress management program has 20 years experience as a certified employee assistance professional. A certified health educator who has worked with diabetes research since 1981 runs the diabetes management program. Therefore, the numerous programs offered and the expertise of the staff makes KC Wellness a top choice in health promotion.

L.L.BEAN, INC.

L.L. Bean is a retail giant with huge catalog sales specializing in outdoor wear, and outdoor equipment. With its headquarters in Freeport, Maine, L.L. Bean first began its health and fitness program in 1982. Since its initiation, the program has grown tremendously as well as comprehensively. Preventive health programs are amongst the most prevalent and important to L.L.Bean. Recognized as a leader, in 1995 the company earned the prestigious C. Everett Koop Award for Workplace Health and Safety. The funding for the health and fitness program comes predominantly from the human resource budget.

L.L.Bean has 15 health and safety professionals' on staff for their employees as well as dependents, retirees, and seasonal employees. Six of these professionals concentrate solely on the health and fitness program. The program was developed through identification of employee needs, a review of scientific literature, and analyzing other programs.

Aside from providing outdoor recreational activities as cross-country skiing and kayaking, L.L. Bean also offers health promotion courses. L.L. Bean even offers a bonus up to $200 for families of employees who participate in prenatal classes, or quit smoking.

The reported goals of the L.L.Bean Employee Health Program are to, "increase overall health, fitness, and related quality of life of employees". A reported example is that they want the employee to be in the 75th percentile of healthiest companies. The first goal is to reduce injuries and illnesses. The second goal is to reduce injury-related loss of work time. The final goal is to reduce health care, workers compensation, disability, and absenteeism cost. The health mission statement for L.L. Bean states as its goal, "to work with area management and employees to achieve and maintain a healthy and safe workplace and promote the health, safety, and fitness of the employees" (LL Bean Health and Fitness Program, 1994).

LL Bean's program focuses on different problems people will encounter in the workplace. Referred to as the "Right Things" to achieve objectives, the first objective is to prevent occupational injury and illness. To achieve this objective, an employee should have an appropriate ergonomic design of workstations and work processes. The employee should have undergone thorough health and safety educational classes and training. The second item the employee should do is work on stretching programs. The third item of this first objective includes using safe industrial hygiene products. The final item would be to reduce other health-related injuries.

The second "Right Things" to achieve objectives includes providing health and fitness programs and fitness assessment to their employees. To achieve this they have five regional fitness centers throughout New England.

L.L. Bean has reported data relating to how their program has helped many employees. This was documented as part of a survey that they gave their employees to ascertain how many of them were taking advantage of the Employee Health Program. The reported percentage of participants is fifty percent. One that is shocking is that only twenty-eight percent use the fitness centers. Twenty-seven percent participate in the health education class. As reported, 68% of L.L. Bean's employees have never had high blood pressure.

METROSPORT ATHLETIC CLUB

MetroSport Athletic Club has over 50,000 square feet of fitness facilities that it offers to other company employees, which includes racquetball courts, and a fitness complex. It is located in Durham, North Carolina, and offers special rates for Duke University employees and students. It is also a partner with Duke's Live for Life Program. Along with the fitness center, MetroSport Athletic Club also has a corporate wellness program that it offers to the employees of other companies. In their corporate wellness program, they offer services and programs including: physiological assessments, exercise prescription, personalized orientation, continued coaching, and the MetroSport Online Magazine. MetroSport also offers a free trial membership. This trial membership allows employees full use of the facility and gives them a chance to become familiar with the club, to acclimate, and determine if they feel comfortable there.

MetroSport also makes appointments with each employee to create a very comprehensive, educational, a thorough fitness program. This orientation session helps the employee become familiar with all of the equipment in the club, and ensures appropriate exercise habits are developed.

Personal training services and additional fitness evaluations can also be purchased through the fitness department. Corporate members can enjoy all the benefits of a regular member, plus an individualized corporate program, which may include: education on healthy lifestyle changes, pre-screening (including body fat testing, and other physiological assessments), and seminars. Motivational programs are available as well as corporate fitness contests, and they may qualify for a reduced membership rate.

MetroSport Athletic Club has been operating since 1983. Since that time, they have come to be recognized as one of the top ranking clubs in the research triangle area. The scope and quality of their health, racquet, swim and fitness complex gives them strengths that makes this an excellent facility. Reportedly, what makes MetroSport's club so appealing is the fact that you won't find better equipment or more qualified, knowledgeable, caring staff anywhere.

MetroSport focuses on helping employees and their families move towards living happier and healthier lifestyles. It is wonderful to know that not only are employees of the company able to use Metrosport and all its facilities, but their family members are also welcome. This is consistent with research that has demonstrated that social support provides assistive mechanisms to increase compliance and adherence to fitness programs.

The certified personal trainers that work at Metrosport have a mission to guide all of their participants to self-improvement. They will work individually with each employee to create an initial personalized fitness program. The personal trainers recognize how important safety is and they make sure that every employee feels safe and comfortable with their health program and their surroundings.

MICHIGAN STATE UNIVERSITY AND THE UNIVERSITY OF MICHIGAN

Both Michigan State University and the University of Michigan have established health promotion programs. Michigan State University (MSU) has a wellness program called the "Healthy U's". "Healthy U's" goal is to create an environment at Michigan State University that supports health. "Healthy U's" provides excellent health promotion programs for all the members of the MSU community. They offer many services that encourage individuals to achieve a healthier, happier, longer life."Health U's" has three "health happens guides" that have helped employees and students immensely. They are listed below:

- Health Happenings Program Guide
- Mayo Health Quest Newsletter
- Well Assured Guides to Better Health

MSU staff has determined that the best way to ascertain how the programs are functioning is through systematic comments and feedback. They post "Healthy U testimonials". They believe this allows individuals to see how others in the program feel about "Healthy U". For example, one participant said, "Healthy U adds a great deal to my working life at MSU." There are many other testimonials that are consistent with these sentiments.

The University of Michigan in Ann Arbor offers a unique wellness program called "M-Fit" Health Promotion. For over 10 years, M-Fit Corporate Health Promotion has been working with employees to help them choose behaviors consistent with healthy lifestyles. This is accomplished by working with employers to develop programs that positively impact not only their employees, but also their organizations. Like most other wellness programs M-Fit's staff will meet with individuals to determine the appropriate level of programming. This is based on individual responses to their questions. Programs are geared to meet the unique needs of each individual. This program was awarded with a silver medal from the Governor's Council on Physical Fitness, Health, and Sports.

The program contains a multitude of services that are open to all employees and certain programs are open to the general public. The services include:

- flu shots
- smoking cessation programs
- stress management programs
- heart health programs
- healthy back programs

- walking and running clubs
- weight management
- fitness consultants
- health risk appraisals
- confidential screenings for depression
- healthy dining programs

The University of Michigan Center for Ergonomics offers a research program that is one of the largest and best known in the United States. Ergonomic studies that assist in workplace design, safety, and injury prevention, are funded by industry, government, and private groups.

MIGRANT FARMER WORKER HEALTH PROGRAM

At the community level of health promotion is a program called the "Camp Health Aide Program" which is coordinated by the Migrant Farm Worker Program in Monroe, Michigan. The goal of Camp Health Aide Program is to, "improve health and wellness to farm working families in the Midwest" (http://monroe. lib.mi.us/cwis/mmhioqfacts.htm). The Camp Health Aide Program has trained 150 male and female migrant farm workers as health promoters since 1985. These men and women provide health education/promotion to their peers in their small farm-working communities using the "Camp Health Aide Manual" which contains many aspects of health and wellness written in both English and Spanish. The Camp Health Aide Program was the 1996 winner of the Models that Work competition, a campaign aimed at increasing access to primary healthcare.

One unique aspect of this program and a probable reason that the Migrant Farm Worker Health Program: Camp Health Aide has been so successful is that the work is being conducted by peers. Individuals that the workers can relate to very well are providing the health promotion programs. Research has demonstrated that advice from a peer, a friend, or a relative may be better received and is less threatening than advice from an unknown professional. The education that the farm workers receive from the "Camp Health Aide Manual" includes topics on Learning Ways of Helping People, Personal Hygiene, Camp Sanitation and Safety, Basic First Aide, Nutrition, Children's Health, Pregnancy, Adult Illness, HIV/AIDS and STD's, Women's Health, and Occupational Health and Safety. These are health topics that will help the workers everyday, and are easily communicable to their peers. Many of the four million migrant farm working families in the U.S. who cannot afford health insurance due to poor wages can significantly benefit from this health promotion program.

NORTHEAST UTILITIES WELLAWARE OUTCOMES

Northeast Utilities, based in Connecticut, employs 6,500 people, and has two million customers. They are New England's largest energy company and a major energy trader in New England. Extensive research on program efficacy and return on investment data is provided and has been organized into five sections for reader clarity.

REDUCED MEDICAL CLAIMS

In 1992, health benefit claims were evaluated to establish benchmark levels of lifestyle and behavioral related costs for Northeast Utilities (NU) population. As a result, WellAware was conceived and implemented during 1994. After 24 months, 1996 claims were analyzed to determine if the WellAware program was producing positive financial results and predict future financial performance. NU experienced flat per capita costs for health care and a $1,200,000 reduction in lifestyle and behavioral claims. Consequentially, the return on investment for the WellAware program, in its first 24 months, was 1:1.6. In other words, for every $1.00 invested $1.60 was saved.

REDUCED HEALTH RISKS

StayWell's HealthPath Health Risk Assessment (HRA), which identifies participant's health risks, is the step to participating in the WellAware Program. The relationship between an increase in the absolute number, and an increase in the severity of health risks, and the corresponding increase in direct medical costs has been demonstrated in published studies.

2,577 participants completed a second HR between 1998-2000. These participant's average lifestyle score improved to 73 compared to 70 at baseline. Individuals also experienced significant reductions in risks, including:

- 31% decrease in smoking
- 29% decrease in lack of exercise
- 16% decrease in mental health risk
- 11% decrease in cholesterol risk
- 10% improvement in eating habits
- 5% decrease in stress

Research has determined that employees with multiple risk factors for heart disease, stroke and psychological and mental health issues, incur much higher average annual medical expenditures that do their lower-risk co-workers.

The percentage of the 2,577, repeat HRA participants with multiple risk factors improved. Participants with:

- fewer than three risk factors increased 6%
- fewer than two risk factors increased 9%
- six or more risk factors decreased 4%

StayWell estimates that these changes have resulted in an annual savings to NU of $1,087,900.

TARGETED INTERVENTION OUTCOMES

Participants, who complete an HRA and are classified as high risk in two or more health areas, were invited to participate in a telephone-based intervention program. The long-term impacts of this intervention model were evaluated in a study. The researchers found that participants in a phone based intervention program were 1) more likely to reduce their risks, than were non-participants; and 2) more likely to reduce their risks in other areas not specially targeted by the intervention. The NU participants who participated in the phone intervention reduced their risk status in all areas, while those who chose to not participate showed an increase in risk levels.

COST SAVINGS FOR INDIVIDUALS WITH CORONARY ARTERY DISEASE

A review of Northeast Utilities 1996 health care claims found that the company experienced total medical costs of $1,377,000 for coronary artery disease (CAD) related claims. Fifty-seven CAD-related hospitalizations resulted in disability plus related impatient costs averaging $46,582 per hospitalization.

Telephone counseling and low cost educational tools (educational materials), have been shown to be effective interventions for disease management. After the implementation of a successful one-year pilot group, a CAD intervention, (consisting of telephone counseling and support materials), was made available to all eligible individuals with diagnosed heart disease. Based on previous NU claims experience, the CAD intervention demonstrated a 72% reduction in all CAD events and a 77% reduction in major CAD events. Improvements in clinical outcomes were demonstrated, as well as a documented high-level of participant satisfaction.

Gross savings were determined by calculating the 12-month anticipated rate of re-hospitalizations versus the actual re-hospitalization rate of NU participants for 12-month time frame. A return on investment of 1:2.6 in reduced medical claims and disability was reported.

SMOKING CESSATION

A smoking cessation intervention was designed based on experts' recommendations for combining behavior modification with the option for drug therapy. Very low cost telephonic counseling was combined with a rebate of $100 for the purchases of approved smoking cessation aids, (Nicotine Patch, Nicotine Inhaler, Zyban, etc.). The 12-month results of this combined intervention resulted in a 44 percent quit rate, with another 12 percent of people stating their intentions to quit. These results far exceed national statistics showing that typical smoking cessation programs achieve a 20 to 30 percent quit rate at six months.

PFIZER

Pfizer is a research based health company that discovers, develops, manufacturers, and markets prescription medicines. Headquartered in New York, New York, it has 90,000 employees, and generates revenue of $32.3 billion. Pzifer makes Viagra, Zoloft, cortisone, Benadryl, Rolaids, Listerine, and Visine.

One of the foremost worksite health promotion programs is Pfizer's Premier Employee Health Promotion Program. Due to the excellence of the program, it was awarded the C.Everett Koop National Health Award in 1999. An ergonomics program within the Premier Employee Health Promotion Program provided the company a 1:3.51 return on investment and saved the 1,033 employees who participated in the program $1.2 million in healthcare costs.

Another money saving program was Pfizer's physical therapy program, which was offered on site at the company's Manhattan NY location. Between 1994 and 1997, 210 employees were given over 3,000 physical therapy sessions. Measured over a time interval, the program generated an average return of investment of 1:2.38, saving the company about $500,000.

The mission and goals for the Premier Employee Health Promotion Program include:

1) to attract and retain the best employees;
2) to develop the most productive and engaged workforce possible;
3) to enhance employee and dependent health by implementing primary, secondary, and tertiary prevention strategies;
4) to effectively manage health care resources, and;
5) to assist employees and dependents to be informed and efficient consumers of health care

These goals are attained due to the great number of services that the program offers. The program components include health risk assessment/identification initiatives, wellness and health education initiatives, disease management initiatives, medical clinics, fitness centers, on-site physical therapy, an ergonomics program, managed disability, welfare benefits, health care delivery evaluation/enhancement, and the employee assistance program.

One reason Pfizer's Premier Employee Health Promotion Program has become a recognized program is the ease in accessing information, and the level of educational support. This provides participants with current information regarding health promotion, and disease risk reduction. The information is communicated to the participants through variety of media including printed pamphlets, and intranet websites. The company also plans many future changes and additions to the program to ensure that it is the best worksite health program available. The changes include using health-risk appraisal data as a diagnostic tool to evaluate health problems, and to periodically repeat the health risk appraisal to provide comparison and to redirect health management efforts. This program allows the spouse and dependents of the employee access to all areas of the program.

The Employee Assistance Program focuses on many issues

within the workforce, including emotional, financial, legal, family, medical, and general work issues. The interest and participation in this program is very high. In the New York site, 85 percent of the employees took part in one or two programs, 80 percent used the on-site health services, and more than 46 percent of the Pfizer workforce participates in the fitness centers.

QUAKER OATS COMPANY

A breakfast food and sports drink corporation, Quaker Oats makes products including Cap'n Crunch and Gatorade. With its headquarters in Chicago, the company was founded in 1901. In 1983, Quaker Oats initiated its health promotion and wellness program. The goal of this program is to lower the health risks of the employees and their families. Quaker Oats is very committed to promoting wellness in its workplace to enhance productivity, decrease absenteeism, enhance productivity, and decrease employee turnover.

Quaker Oats is the only company to win the Wellness Council of America's "Gold Well Workplace Award" for quality and excellence in corporate health promotion programming three years (1992, 1996, and 1999. Note: this award is not given each year). Notable entities include the highly acclaimed Gatorade Sports Science Institute, which conducts research, and provides education in sports nutrition, exercise science, and sports medicine.

The health promotion and wellness program consist primarily of three elements. First is the "Live Well-Be-Well" program, which provides intervention for the employees. Through these interventions, coordinated by Corporate Health Services, employees and their families learn about stress management, weight management, healthy back care, and various other health-related topics.

The second component is the "Quaker Flex Benefit" plan. This plan provides financial incentives for up to $500.00 per family each year for making lifestyle pledges. The lifestyle pledges include: 1) car seats and seatbelts when driving; 2) participating in at least 20 minutes of aerobic exercise at least three times a week; and 3) no use of tobacco products in the last six months and no use of them in the future. There are also other opportunities to earn money by completing health-risk appraisals, screenings, and making lifestyle pledges. The health risk appraisal includes screening for cholesterol, blood pressure, and weight. If a risk factor value or classification falls outside the recommended and accepted levels, intervention steps are taken.

The third component to health and wellness promotion program at Quaker Oats is an educational program entitled "Informed Choices". Through group meetings and lectures, employees and their families learn how to efficiently ask questions of their health care provider. The program also provides hospital pricing data, and consumer-orientated publications.

The fitness center is one of the features of Quaker's "Live Well-Be-Well" health promotion program. The fitness center provides the opportunity to improve flexibility, strength, endurance, and cardiovascular fitness through exercise. Personal lifestyle counseling regarding nutrition, weight, and stress management is available. A second feature is health services which helps prevent and/or detect early health risks, and provides good examples of primary and secondary prevention efforts.

Quaker's employee assistance program assists employees and eligible family members in finding alternatives, and assistance with interpersonal problems. Their health resource center is a service that promotes self-learning, and supports the concept that individual employees can make a difference in managing their own health.

REGIS UNIVERSITY

Regis University, located in Denver, Colorado, developed a wellness program for the students called "Life Directions". The university's wellness philosophy states that each of us must learn about the physical, psychological, spiritual, career, social, and intellectual dimensions of our daily lives. The belief is that students can benefit through coordinated wellness programs whose purpose is to educate and offer skills in making lifestyle choices and behavioral changes. The Life Directions program offers educational programs through campus departments including: counseling, career services, student health services, the fitness center, wellness programs, as well as disability services.

The university's Life Directions program offers a variety of activities. Personal counseling offers psychological assessments and referrals as well as educational workshops and stress management classes. General information is provided to parents about common issues college students face such as: adult children of alcohol, anger, eating disorders, sleeping disorders, suicide prevention, and trauma. If a student is facing any of the aforementioned issues, individual counseling, psychological assessments, referrals, crisis intervention, education workshops, stress management, and collaborative care with health services is available.

Regis University's wellness program provides prevention classes such as: substance abuse prevention, smoking cessation program, reasons to quit smoking and "why do I smoke". Regis also offers health resources and information on various health related topics. These include personal fitness plans, fitness fundamentals, nutrition tips, dietary guidelines, nutritional analyses, body mass index (BMI) measurements, and body fat assessments.

The mission of the health promotion program at Regis focuses on holistic education. The behavioral health promotion program addresses these needs by offering programs and services designed to encompass the six dimensions of wellness. These are physical, mental, emotional, social, communal, and spiritual. The health promotion programs are nutrition and fitness, healthy relationships, stress management, and "entering a stress free zone". The programs are designed to target traditional undergraduate students, but can easily be adapted to work with adult students, and staff.

Regis' harm prevention program is designed to minimize potential hazards by addressing high-risk behavior and environmental vulnerabilities. The behavioral health program addresses concerns about substance abuse through general prevention campaigns, and programs targeting high-risk groups through personalized interventions for high-risk individuals. Violence prevention addresses hate crimes, rape, and physical assaults.

The leaders at Regis University believe that all of the programs listed above will foster the concept of wellness and will help the students make healthy choices, and positive changes. Regis University believes that these programs will help create better morale, less absenteeism, better productivity, and overall positive health benefits.

SANTA CLARA COUNTY WELLNESS PROGRAM

Santa Clara County of California has developed an employee wellness program that is offered to all county employees in many county locations.

The wellness mission statement of Santa Clara County states, "The employee wellness program is dedicated to enhancing the health and well being of Santa Clara County employees by providing services that motivate employees to move toward optimal health. Improved health of an employee can lead to increased productivity, improved morale, decreased incidence of accidents and injuries, and decreased medical costs and absenteeism".

The goals of Santa Clara employee wellness program are to provide worksite health promotion services that are easily accessible to as many employees as possible, and to provide services and programs that motivate people to learn new skills, and make positive lifestyle changes.

The Santa Clara County wellness programs are staffed and supervised by trained health professionals. Employee participation in this wellness program is voluntary and confidential.

The Santa Clara wellness program provides a wide range of services such as: fitness assessments, screening services, health appraisals, a quarterly newsletter, a lending library, and health education information. Also individual consultations regarding health and wellness are available, as well as, onsite nurse hours at selected sites, sponsorships of activity programs to promote fitness, yoga, and tai chi classes.

Screening services include blood pressure, cholesterol, glucose, bone density, and pulmonary function. Employees receive a free consultation followed by a thorough review by a health care professional. Fitness assessments include testing for strength, flexibility, and cardiovascular fitness. Participants complete a health risk questionnaire before beginning a fitness program. Recommendations are provided two weeks after the assessment. Health risk appraisals include a computerized summary of individual's health based on information provided by participant. A newsletter called "Wellness Works" is distributed four times a year with the newest research findings and tips for good health. The lending library for the employee wellness program contains books, pamphlets, videos, and audiotapes on a variety of health and wellness topics.

Classes are offered for employee development and by departmental request to meet the needs of individual work groups. A variety of classes are offered including: parenting, building stretching, and strengthening into your exercise routine, neck and back care, low fat cooking, smoking cessation, C.P.R., healthy living with chronic conditions, and managing cardiovascular risk factors. Chair massage is a unique service that is offered in the work place to relieve the neck, back, and arm pain that accompanies stress.

Classes offered include: "Awareness at Work", "Dynamics of Diabetes", "Nutrition for a Healthier You", "C.P.R. For Family And Friends", "New Cooking Ideas for Eating Well", "Women's Health Issues In The Middle Years: Forty And Forward", and "Building Better Bones".

"Awareness At Work" is a program that teaches individuals how to better handle stress, and can improve a person's ability to solve workplace problems. This program also teaches effective skills for dealing with job stress, boosting patience and tolerance in complex situations, and increasing the capacity to listen and empathize with others. "Dynamics of Diabetes" is a comprehensive course that addresses the principles of diabetes mellitus, medications, blood glucose self-monitoring, and signs, symptoms and treatment for hypoglycemia or hyperglycemia. A certified diabetes educator teaches this class as well as a nutrition class called "Nutrition For A Healthier You". This class presents the new nutritional guidelines for diabetes and additional general nutrition. The class focuses on the effects of food on blood sugar, serving sizes for weight loss, blood sugar control, label reading, and carbohydrate counting.

"Women's Health Issues In The Middle Years: Forty And Forward" is a workshop designed to provide an overview of women's changing physical, emotional, and sexual lives from premenopause through menopause. A registered nurse and a family nurse practitioner facilitate this workshop. Topics include natural hormones, phyto-hormones, wild yam extract, herbal medicine, risks and benefits of hormone replacement therapy, nutrition, vitamin supplements, breast cancer, and heart disease. "Building Better Bones" is a class offered as an osteoporosis management class. Employees learn about causes, risk factors, and foods rich in calcium. They also learn which medications are used for treatment and how to interpret a bone density report.

These classes and services contribute to an effective wellness program for the county and help people attain their personal health goals.

SC JOHNSON WAX

SC Johnson Wax is a large consumer chemical company that produces home cleaners, bug sprays, and a newly introduced product "Saran Cutting Strips". Armstrong Park located in Racine, Wisconsin is a corporate entity and private preserve for 2,700 employees at the headquarters of SC Johnson Wax.

The fitness center and recreational areas are part of a conscientious proactive business strategy by the company to maintain health care cost stability by helping employees maintain good health and fitness. The park is located eight miles from the headquarters that includes employees of both offices and the manufacturing plant. Armstrong Park sits on 146 acres with walking and running trails, an aquatics center and a recreational center. This includes a gymnasium, an Olympic-sized indoor pool, strength training equipment, an aerobic exercise studio, hot tubs, massage service, meeting rooms, and a video library.

The grounds of the facility include a pair of softball fields, a golf driving range, tennis and volleyball courts, an archery range, horseshoe pits, playgrounds, and picnic areas.

Guided by a health promotion coordinator, fitness classes are offered as well as healthy eating plans. Every year there is a fitness challenge competition, with points and prizes for regularly exercising, quitting smoking, and losing weight.

In the Milwaukee area, an overweight employee who smokes costs a company from $500.00 - $800.00 a year more than a nonsmoking, recommended healthy weight employee. An internal research analysis reported that SC Johnson Wax spent $5,587 per employee or retiree for health care in 1993-1994, 15% *less* than it had in 1991-1992. This is a very positive result in an environment of escalating health care costs.

UNIVERSITY OF RHODE ISLAND

The University of Rhode Island, with a student population of 14,000, has a health promotion program known as "URI Fitness/Wellness". This program is, "designed to help the individual improve cardiovascular fitness, increase muscular strength and endurance, improve flexibility, and become better educated on fitness and wellness issues" (www.uri.edu). This program achieves its goals through the use of fitness programs, exercise testing, personal training (provided by certified personal trainers), a fitness center, and wellness workshops. The fitness programs offered include "Hard Bodies" (non-cardiovascular), "20/20/20" (low-impact aerobics, step, and conditioning), Tae Bo, "Cardio Zone" (high impact cardiovascular exercises and muscle toning with free weights), yoga, Tae Kwan Do, and many more. The fitness testing offered includes a sub-maximal cardiovascular assessment as well as measurements of muscular endurance, girth measurements, resting heart rate, body compositions, and blood pressure. The wellness workshops are offered each month and include "Strength Labs" which focus on specific muscle groups and provide information on technique and effectiveness, and "Changes for a Healthier Body" which incorporates safe and effective methods to begin a healthy weight loss programs. The URI Fitness/Wellness programs are available for students of the URI community as well as non-students.

US DEPARTMENT OF HEALTH AND HUMAN SERVICES: CENTER FOR DISEASE CONTROL AND PREVENTION

The United States Department of Health and Human Services (USDHHS) Center for Disease Control and Prevention is a government entity that offers and promotes many different types of health promotion programs across the country.

One of these programs is The National Skin Cancer Prevention and Education Program. The goal of this program is to achieve the *Healthy People 2010* skin cancer prevention goals. These goals aim at increasing the percentage of people who regularly use at least one protective measure, limit sun exposure and wear sunscreen from 47% to 75% of all adults. The goals also include increasing skin cancer awareness and prevention behaviors among all populations, particularly those at high risk, and developing and supporting partnerships to extend and reinforce skin care messages for behavior change. Additional goals include coordinating nationwide efforts to reduce skin cancer incidence and death, and developing a national skin cancer prevention and education plan. The Center for Disease Control (CDC) was successful at reaching the public in 2001 using an advertising campaign called *"Choose Your Cover"*. The campaign utilized television and radio public service announcements, posters, brochures, and a web site. The *"Choose Your Cover"* campaign emphasized that skin cancer is a largely preventable disease. A pamphlet distributed by the CDC for the campaign discusses of the burdens of skin cancer. It stresses that malignant melanoma, the most rapidly increasing form of cancer in the United States, causes more than 75% of all deaths from skin cancer. It further emphasizes that malignant melanoma diagnosed at an early stage can usually be cured, but melanoma diagnosed at late stage is more likely to spread and cause death (www.cdc.gov). In the same publication, the CDC lists who is at risk for developing skin cancer. Among those listed were individuals with fair to light skin complexion, a positive family history of skin cancer, and freckles. The main part of this pamphlet was the prevention section. Five brightly colored pictures with captions reading; *"Get a Hat", "Seek the Shade", "Cover Up", "Rub it On",* and *"Get Shades"* were highlighted. An easy and fun way to get the message out to a wide audience was created. The CDC also funds different skin cancer prevention demonstrations that promote safe sun habits. These programs include *"Pool Cool"* which is implemented at public swimming pools across the country, and *"Sunwise Stampede"* which has been implemented at the San Diego Zoo. Also, *"The National Coalition for Skin Cancer Prevention in Health, Physical Education, Recreation, and Youth Sports"* which provides prevention education to professionals who work in youth sports programs, parks and recreation programs, and elementary and middle school health education, and *"The Coalition for Skin Cancer Prevention in Maryland"*. The USDHHS and the CDC also offer a multitude of programs, and services in many other health related areas, from "Aging" to "Zoontonic Diseases".

WORLD HEALTH ORGANIZATION

The World Health Organization (WHO) originated on April 7, 1948 with the objective of helping all people attain maximal health and wellness. This organization, coordinated by the United Nations, is able to accomplish this goal by funding a plethora of health promotion programs on all heath topics imaginable. The WHO health promotion programs include the *Global Program for the*

Prevention & Control of Rheumatic Heart Disease, Diabetes Awareness Program, HIV/Aids Programs, and many more.

One service is the World Health Organization's *Diabetes Awareness Program* that is responsible for providing all members of the WHO (190 Countries) advice on appropriate policies and strategies for monitoring, prevention and control of diabetes. The WHO believes that diabetes poses a great health risk that for many years has gone under recognized. They believe that if the current rise in diabetes continues, the prevalence of the disorder will more than double from 140 million to 300 million in the next 25 years. The WHO has set up Diabetes Collaborating centers in nine countries around the world (including the U.S.) that specialize in the development of appropriate technology for the control of diabetes, and the study and control of the long term complications of the disorder, as well as many other associated areas. The WHO is doing all it can to provide education about diabetes, and to implement effective prevention strategies to combat the effects of this widespread disorder.

CONCLUSION

Throughout this comprehensive review, it was consistently demonstrated that the health promotion and wellness programs have similar goals and mission statements to incorporate primary, secondary, and tertiary preventive efforts through both preventive care, and lifestyle management. The programs are primarily dedicated to the participant's overall health and wellness.

Existing programs, large and small, in private as well as public facilities were included in the review. Multinational organizations, public and private universities, and programs within the community were provided for comparison. Businesses that provide health promotion and wellness services for other organizations were also included. Awards were noted to recognize the prestige and value these programs have attained at the state, and national level.

The programs reviewed concentrated their efforts on the different dimensions of wellness by offering educational and awareness programs, screenings, and services in fitness and health, spiritual, emotional, environmental, intellectual, psychological, and social health. In many instances, individualized programs were available based upon personal as well as organizational needs, interests, and a variety of physiological and psychological health assessments. Employee assistance programs were included and are recognized as a partner in efforts to produce a healthier workforce. A highly qualified and trained staff is employed to assist with program development, implementation, and evaluation.

The leaders of these entities, businesses, and organizations believe that the implementation of health promotion and wellness programs will create environments conducive to improved morale, less absenteeism, increased productivity, and generally, foster overall positive health benefits. Health promotion and wellness programs may be able to reduce the demand for medical services, decrease workplace injuries, and subsequently worker compensation costs. By employing preventive and proactive health promotion and wellness measures, the bottom-line objective is to help lower the escalating costs associated with health care.

The return on investment data and statistical analyses of health promotion and wellness programming demonstrates the inherent concern for positive results. Research studies, and the extensive data analyses are specifically designed to document financial efficacy. Decreasing the number and severity of primary risk factors, and specifically targeting high-risk population groups (i.e. the employees with severe hypercholesterolemia) through prevention, active intervention, and education was shown to produce a valid return on investment.

There are numerous benefits associated with the implementation of health promotion and wellness programs, including physiological and psychological benefits that can translate into increased productivity, improved morale, reduced absenteeism, and overall improved job performance. It is a hope that employer sponsored wellness and health promotion programs in the workplace will help build a strong foundation of healthy, and productive employees.

CHAPTER EIGHT

RESEARCH AND DATA ANALYSIS OF A SELECTED HEALTH PROMOTION PROGRAM

The previous chapter introduced and thoroughly analyzed a multitude of existing health promotion programs and detailed integral program components, leadership and staff, and documented return on investment data or financial efficacy. This chapter specifically focuses on one employee based health promotion program, details specific program components, and explores intervention strategies that produce physiological efficacy.

The University of Wisconsin at Stevens Point implemented the first university based employee wellness program in 1986.[1] Slippery Rock University (PA) implemented its wellness program also in 1986, and according to a survey by the National Wellness Institute, about 20% of higher education institutions had employee wellness programs in 1986.[2] Between 1986-1992, the prevalence of employee wellness programs grew another 15% and by 1992, 35% of universities had established programs.[3]

Slippery Rock University (SRU) is one of 14 state-owned institutions that comprise the State System of Higher Education of the Commonwealth of Pennsylvania. According to a comprehensive survey completed by Caler, one-half of the 14 universities within this system have established programs. While this percentage may seem low, it met the objective as established in Healthy People 2000.[4-5]

While SRU was the first university in the Pennsylvania State System of Higher Education to implement a wellness program, all seven programs were implemented between 1986-1995. The most common programs offered include percent body fat and weight measurements, blood pressure, cholesterol and glucose screenings, which are offered at one-half of universities that sponsor a program. Fitness programs including assessments of strength, flexibility, and cardiovascular efficiency are offered at approximately one-third of the universities that offer programs. Since the purpose of this study was to assess the prevalence of employer sponsored health promotion programs in the State System of Higher Education, specific information related to the intervention component of the programs was not included in the study. According to the survey, most of the implemented programs are annually evaluated for participant satisfaction; however, the program at SRU is the only program to provide statistical evidence of program efficacy.[4]

INTRODUCTION TO THE RESEARCH AND DATA ANALYSIS

The purpose of this chapter is to thoroughly investigate the effects of one university based employee health promotion program on twelve physiological parameters of health related to cardiovascular disease, and to document physiological efficacy. The physiological variables have been quantified and collectively are termed a cardiovascular disease risk profile. A second objective of this analysis is to investigate the specific influence of exercise on the cardiovascular disease risk profiles by assessing profile differences between active and non-active subjects at entry into the health promotion program, and by investigating how an increase in exercise duration affected the variables used to quantify the cardiovascular disease risk profile. Cardiovascular disease risk profiles were quantified through an assessment of cardiovascular fitness (estimated VO_2max), systolic and diastolic blood pressure, percent body fat, body mass index (BMI), weight, and serum lipid levels of total cholesterol (TC), high density lipoproteins (HDL), low density lipoproteins (LDL), the ratio of TC to HDL, and the level of serum glucose. A cardiovascular disease risk profile included clinical measurements of: (a) cardiovascular efficiency, systolic and diastolic blood pressure, estimated percent body fat, body mass index, and total body weight; and (b) a lipid profile of total cholesterol, high density lipoproteins, low density lipoproteins, the ratio of total cholesterol to high density lipoproteins, and serum glucose. Five research hypotheses were investigated to determine and assess program efficacy. They are listed below:

1. At the conclusion of the sixteen-week employee based health promotion program, the variables used to quantify the cardiovascular disease risk profile will improve.
2. At entry, there will be a significant difference between the cardiovascular disease risk profiles of pre-program exercisers and pre-program non-exercisers.
3. There will be a significant difference between the cardiovascular disease risk profiles of subjects who increase exercise and subjects who do not increase exercise.
4. There will be a significant difference between the cardiovascular disease risk profiles of pre-program exercisers who increase exercise and pre-program exercisers who do not increase exercise.

5. There will be a significant difference between the cardiovascular disease risk profiles of pre-program non-exercisers who increase exercise and pre-program non-exercisers who do not increase exercise.

RESEARCH METHODOLOGY

The purpose of this section is to describe the research methodology employed in this study and for that purpose this section has been divided into the following sections: (a) information on the testing environment, testing instrumentation, measurement procedures and clinical measures; (b) program and intervention components; (c) selection of subjects; (d) research design and research variables; and, (e) treatment of the data.

INFORMATION ON THE TESTING ENVIRONMENT, TESTING INSTRUMENTATION, MEASUREMENT PROCEDURES, AND CLINICAL MEASURES

The procedures used to assess the physiological parameters measured in this study have been examined, and for the purpose of this study, the following procedures were implemented. In accordance with the recommendations of the American College of Sports Medicine, the testing environment was maintained at a temperature of between 70 and 74 degrees Fahrenheit. The assessment procedures were explained prior to initiating the test and each subject completed the fitness center membership application, medical history, and informed consent for exercise testing and exercise prescription.

The information collected during the assessment was recorded on the assessment form and each subject was given the following instructions prior to the physiological assessment:

1. Refrain from ingesting food, alcohol, or caffeine three hours prior to the assessment.
2. Avoid significant exertion on the day of the assessment.

3. Wear comfortable clothing that permits freedom of movement.
4. Subjects were advised to adhere to their standard medication schedule.
5. Subjects were advised to bring a list of medications to the assessment, including dosage, frequency, and a record of the time the last dose was taken. This medication information was recorded on the assessment form.

In accordance with the guidelines of the American College of Sports Medicine, the physiological assessments were performed in the following order: (a) age; (b) height; (c) weight; (d) resting heart rate; (e) resting blood pressure; (f) percent body fat - skinfold measurements (abdomen, ilium, and triceps); (g) submaximal ergometer test; (h) body mass index (BMI); and, (i) the blood profile (assessed on a separate day).

The following procedures were followed during each assessment. The assessments were completed at entry into the program, and at the completion of the 16-week intervention program.

1. Standing height. This measurement was made with the Detecto Physician scale stadiometer while the subject was wearing socks. The participant stood with the heels together, then stretched upward to the fullest extent. The heels, buttocks, and upper back were straight and the chin was not lifted. The measurement was recorded to the nearest 0.25 of an inch.

2. Weight. This measurement was made using the Detecto Physician scale while the subject was wearing light clothes (t-shirt, shorts) and no shoes. The scale was calibrated prior to each measurement. The weight was recorded to the nearest quarter of a pound.

3.   Resting heart rate. Prior to the measurement, the subject was instructed to rest quietly in a chair for five minutes. The measurement was made by palpation of the radial pulse for 30 seconds and multiplied by two to arrive at a one minute resting heart rate value.

4.   Resting blood pressure. This measurement was made immediately following the resting heart rate measurement while the individual was sitting upright in a straight-backed chair with both feet flat on the floor and with the left arm flexed and resting on a table. The blood pressure was measured with a mercury sphygmomanometer (manufactured by PyMaH Corporation, Summerville, NJ) and a Gold Accent Professional stethoscope. The adjustable blood pressure cuff, manufactured by PyMaH Corporation was placed on the upper left arm at approximately heart level. The column was positioned as close as possible to eye level in order to reduce parallax error. The proper size cuff was used (obese or adult) because having a cuff that is too small will overestimate blood pressure. The cuff was inflated to 200 mmHg (above where Korotkoff sounds are no longer heard) and the stethoscope was placed in the antecubital space below the cuff. The cuff was inflated to 220 mmHg during the exercise portion of the assessment. The test administrator began to deflate the cuff slowly at about three mmHg per second. The appearance of the first distinct tapping sound was recorded as the systolic blood pressure reading. The sounds become louder at first, then began to fade. The disappearance of the tapping sounds was recorded as the diastolic pressure.

If more than one reading was to be made, a few minutes were allowed for normal circulation to return to the arm. If the sounds were not clear and sharp, they were amplified by opening and clenching the fist five or six times while the arm was raised and then the procedures were started again. The examiner was instructed to refrain from pressing too hard on the stethoscope, as this could have contributed to an erroneously low diastolic reading.[6]

5. Percent body fat assessment. The three-site skinfold test for both men and women was utilized. The sites for both genders were the abdomen, ilium, and the triceps. All measurements were made on the right side of the subject using a Lange skinfold caliper (Cambridge Scientific Industries, Cambridge, MD). The test administrator determined the location of the skinfold. The subcutaneous tissue was grasped firmly between the thumb and index finger of the left hand and separated or pulled away from the muscle tissue. The amount pinched was enough to form a fold with parallel sides. The skinfold caliper was held in the right hand perpendicular to the skinfold with the dial facing up. The caliper heads were placed 0.25 of an inch away from the fingers holding the skinfold. The caliper dial was read four seconds after placing the caliper on the skinfold. A constant pressure was maintained between the thumb and forefinger at all times. Fifteen seconds were allotted between measurements.

The abdomen measurement is a horizontal skinfold located one inch to the right of and one-half inch below the naval. The ilium is a diagonal skinfold located at the top of the iliac crest on the mid-axillary line. The triceps measurement is a vertical skinfold located mid-way between the acromion process and the inferior portion of the elbow on the rear midline of the arm. The arm remained extended and relaxed throughout the measurements.

Three measurements were made at each site. If any measure varied by more than 0.5 mm, a fourth measurement was taken and used. The mean of three measurements was computed and was used to determine percent body fat.

6. Cardiovascular assessment. The submaximal cardiovascular assessment was performed on a Monark Ergometer, model 818E manufactured by Monark AB in Sweden. The instrument was calibrated each fall prior to the physiological assessments according to the instruction manual. The YMCA submaximal ergometer test, used to assess peak oxygen uptake and predict maximum work capacity was utilized.[7] The following procedures were followed.

The metronome was set at 100 beats per minute and each subject pedaled the ergometer at a rate of 50 revolutions per minute. A three to five minute warm-up phase preceded the data collection. There was no tension during the warm-up stage. At the completion of the warm-up, the first workload was set at 0.5 kp.

Each stage of the test lasted from between three and four minutes, depending on the willingness of the subject, heart rate, blood pressure, and related physiological responses. During the last ten seconds of the second and third minutes (and fourth minute, if necessary) of each stage, the radial pulse was palpated for ten seconds, multiplied by six, and recorded as the exercising heart rate. If the measured heart rates varied by more than five beats per minute between the second and third minute of the stage, a fourth minute was added and the heart rate measured.

In accordance with the YMCA test procedures, a pulse dependent workload chart was utilized to determine stage progression.[7] After a warm-up of three to four minutes with no ergometer tension, the initial workload was set according to the gender of the subject. In order to attain a more linear heart rate response, the second workload was set to 1.5 kp and progressed 0.5 kp every stage thereafter. If the subjects' heart rate exceeded 100 beats per minute during the first stage, the second workload was maintained at 1.0 kp with an increase of 0.5 kp every stage thereafter. The objective of the YMCA submaximal bicycle test is to obtain two heart rates between 110 and 150 beats per minute. The test is designed to attain linear heart rate responses and achieve a cardiovascular steady state in order to assess a heart rate response at a specific workload. When two workloads provided a heart rate response of between 110-150 beats per minute, the test was terminated. A cool-down phase of three to four minutes or until the heart rate response fell below 100 beats per minute followed. The blood pressure measurements were taken between the second and third minutes of each stage and at the termination of the test.

In accordance with the guidelines of the American College of Sports Medicine, if specific conditions arise, the test was terminated immediately. Included in the termination criteria were angina, a 20 mmHg drop in systolic blood pressure or failure of systolic blood pressure to rise with increased workloads, excessive rise in systolic blood pressure greater than 220 mmHg or diastolic pressure greater than 110 mmHg, lightheadedness, confusion, cyanosis, and nausea. Also, termination criteria included failure of the heart rate to increase with an increase in workload, physical manifestations of severe fatigue, or if the subject requested to stop.

The data were recorded on the assessment form and MetCalc Software was used to calculate VO_2 max in ml/kg/min.[8] After the calculation of relative maximal oxygen consumption, the value was multiplied by 1000. This product was divided by the subject's weight in kilograms to attain the subjects absolute maximal oxygen consumption recorded in liters per minute (l/m).

7.   Body Mass Index (BMI): Quetelet Index. The Quetelet Index is the most widely accepted test of BMI.[6] The calculated indices can be used to represent different body composition classifications. A subject's Quetelet Index is determined by dividing their weight in kilograms by the square of their height in meters and is recorded as kg/m^2. The MetCalc Software program was used to calculate BMI.

8.   Blood profile. The blood profile assessment consisted of a measurement of total cholesterol (TC), low density lipoproteins (LDL), high density lipoproteins (HDL), the ratio of TC to HDL cholesterol, and a measurement of blood glucose. All measurements were recorded in milligrams per deciliter (mg/dl). The instrument that was used to assess total cholesterol and HDL cholesterol was the Paramax Total Cholesterol Reagent, manufactured by Dade International Inc. The Paramax Cholesterol Reagent formulation is based on a modification of the method of Allain et al.[9]

> Cholesterol esterase catalyzes the hydrolysis of   .
> cholesterol esters to free cholesterol. The cholesterol is
> oxidized by atmospheric oxygen in the presence of
> cholesterol oxidase to hydrogen peroxide and cholest-4-
> en-3-one. In the presence of peroxidase, the hydrogen

peroxide formed oxidatively couples with 4-aminoantipyrine and 3,5-dichloro-2-hydroxy benzene sulfonic acid, sodium salt, to yield a chromogen which is monitored bichromatically at 525/630 nm. For the determination of HDL cholesterol, the reaction is preceded by isoelectric-polyanionic precipitation of low-density lipoproteins (Dade International Inc, 1995).

Validation studies on the Paramax Cholesterol procedure report a correlation coefficient of 0.984 for total cholesterol and a correlation coefficient of 0.988 for HDL cholesterol. Calibration of the Paramax Analyzer was in accordance with the operator's manual.

LDL cholesterol was calculated from the measurement of TC utilizing the standard equation:

$$LDL - C = TC - (HDL)/5 - Triglycerides^{1}$$

The Paramax Glucose Reagent was used to assess blood glucose values. The Paramax Glucose Reagent is a modification of the coupled enzymatic method of Slein.[10]

The modifications involve the use of NAD+ rather than NADP+ and glucose-6-phosphate dehydrogenase from Leuconostoc mesenteroides rather than yeast. Glucose is phosphorylated to glucose-6-phosphate in the presence of hexokinase converted to 6-phosphogloconate in the presence of G-6-PDH, and NAD+ is reduced to NADH causing a change in absorbance that is monitored bichromatically at 340/405 nm (Dade International, 1995).

Validation studies on the Paramax glucose procedure report a correlation coefficient of 0.997. Calibration of the Paramax

---

[1] provided triglycerides are less than 400 mg/dl

Analyzer was in accordance with the operator's manual. The ratio of TC to HDL cholesterol was calculated from the appropriate measurements.

Subjects were advised to refrain from exercising, eating and drinking 12 hours prior to the test. Water consumption was permissible.

PROGRAM AND INTERVENTION COMPONENTS

Slippery Rock University is one of 14 state-owned institutions that comprise the State System of Higher Education of the Commonwealth of Pennsylvania. Integral to its mission is the development of programs and services to foster a healthy campus environment for its employees. A primary dimension of the university's efforts to promote health is an employee wellness program. The Slippery Rock University Employee Wellness Program is a multi-faceted, educationally based health promotion program for the faculty and staff. Program objectives focus on improving morale, productivity, internal communication, improving and increasing the awareness of the benefits of a healthy lifestyle, and reducing health care costs to the university.

Implemented in the fall semester of 1986, the wellness program has served over 400 employees. The program lasts 16 weeks (one semester) and is structured specifically to provide individualized attention to each participant. The program consists of two components: knowledge and intervention. The knowledge component contains a multitude of services that are provided and available free of charge to all program participants. The standardized services include nutrition education and dietary analysis, and video-taped presentations on all aspects of health, including nutrition, cardiovascular fitness, coronary artery disease, exercise programs, exercising under various environmental conditions, body composition and weight control, and smoking cessation. Also, a consumer video that provides valuable information on how to choose foods correctly and how to read food labels is available. Numerous research articles, fliers, brochures and pamphlets and a faculty/staff newsletter, "The Wright Workout", are also distributed.

The intervention component is comprised of an individualized wellness and exercise prescription that is based on the results of preliminary physiological and cognitive inventories. The wellness prescription is tailored to specifically meet the needs of the individual. The exercise component of the intervention program follows the guidelines of the American College of Sports Medicine. Participants exercise three to five times per week for a duration of at least 20 minutes (up to 60 minutes) at an intensity level of 60-80% of their age-adjusted maximal heart rate. Exercise intensity is also monitored using a rating of perceived exertion. Following the scale developed by Gunnar Borg, participants are instructed to maintain an exercise intensity of "fairly light" to "somewhat hard", a corresponding number of 11-14. Aerobic conditioning exercises are emphasized and are supplemented with resistance exercises.

Subjects reported to the fitness center at least three times per week at one of three preferred times (6:00 - 8:00 a.m., 11:00 a.m. - 1:00 p.m. or 4:00 - 6:00 p.m.). Each subject was given a 60-minute orientation to the facility and equipment. Prior to the orientation, the director of the fitness center prepared an exercise prescription. Included in the exercise prescription were flexibility exercises, cardiovascular conditioning parameters, muscular strength and endurance guidelines and information on warm up and cool down activities. Subjects were given a workout card to record duration, intensity, and modality of cardiovascular conditioning, along with sets, repetitions, and weight on resistance machines.

Prior to initiating the exercise session, subjects performed flexibility exercises and a five-minute warm up. Cardiovascular training preceded muscular strength and endurance conditioning. A cool down phase was monitored and each individual continued to exercise at a diminishing intensity until the heart rate fell below 100 beats per minute.

Modalities available to develop cardiovascular fitness included treadmills, stairmasters, bicycle ergometer (recumbent, air-dynes and windracers), cross-country ski simulators, rowers, versa-climbers, a stepmill, and a variety of aerobic dance classes. Participants were given an individual orientation on each piece, and directed to use a modality (or modalities) that reflected and suited their medical history, assessment results, program goals, and exercise preferences. Individuals with pre-existing conditions or conditions that would necessitate or restrict specific modalities were directed to use the recommended modality (or modalities).

Resistance exercises were employed using a variety of strength training equipment including Cybex, Nautilus, York dumbbells, and hand weights. The aerobic dance classes incorporated resistance work with the use of hand weights, and resistance tubing. In accordance with the guidelines of the American College of Sports Medicine, the participants performed one set of between 8 and 12 repetitions at 60% of one repetition maximum on each piece of equipment. An individual program was designed incorporating specific program goals, medical history, assessment results, and exercise preferences. Gradual progression of the aerobic and resistance training sessions was accomplished through weekly participant meetings and observations.

The pre-program inventories consisted of a comprehensive physiological assessment, a three-day dietary analysis, and a five-component blood profile. The physiological assessment included measurements of resting and exercising heart rate and blood pressure, height, weight, body composition (skinfold measurements), muscular strength and muscular endurance, flexibility and a sub-maximal cardiovascular assessment. The five component blood profile measured total cholesterol (TC), HDL, LDL, and glucose values. The ratio of TC to HDL was also calculated.

The cognitive inventories consisted of a comprehensive health risk appraisal – The Lifestyle Assessment Questionnaire (5th edition LA-Q), and written information about each individual's medical history, exercise preferences, program goals, along with a signed informed consent.

The pre-program assessments were completed and the results were presented at a "Kick-off Breakfast", with the president and other administrators of the university, and the members of the employee wellness committee. Throughout the semester, the members of the wellness committee were available to provide feedback, answer questions, help interpret data, and to offer encouragement and support for the newest members of the wellness program. Each participant in the employee wellness program was given a free semester membership to the fitness center, as well as a wellness program t-shirt, a water bottle, and at the completion of the program a gym bag, and a certificate of participation.

During the 16 weeks, the participants were targeted to receive specific information based on the results of their preliminary physiological and cognitive inventories, their interests and program goals. Employees who had elevated blood lipid profile values were given information and provided feedback on all aspects of nutrition and strategies to reduce blood lipid values. The program also serves as an avenue of primary prevention. Through pre-program screenings, some pre-existing conditions were exposed (i.e. hypertension, abnormal physiological responses to the sub-maximal cardiovascular assessment). In this instance, participants were referred to the appropriate health care provider for follow-up care. Depending on the severity of the condition and the professional recommendations of both the health care provider and the director of the fitness center, the subject may have continued in the program. Although the program functions on a limited budget, it is reported to be highly effective primarily because of the personalized and individualized attention given to each participant. Early intervention and appropriate follow-up are keys to the effectiveness of the program.

After the 16 weeks, each participant was given a post-program physiological assessment in order to determine the effectiveness of the program. To motivate and encourage the participants to continue a healthy lifestyle after participation in the wellness program a reduced rate to join the fitness center was provided.

SELECTION OF SUBJECTS

This study included data taken from the physiological assessments of subjects who participated in the employee wellness program (EWP) at Slippery Rock University (SRU). One hundred and fifty-four subjects, 61 men and 93 women, between the ages of 25-60 years participated in this study. Subjects completed the pre-program inventories, the 16-week intervention program, and the post-program assessments. Complete data sets per physiological variable were used to quantify the cardiovascular disease risk profile. Information obtained from the Office of Affirmative Action indicates that Slippery Rock University employs 800 full-time people in a variety of executive, administrative, management, faculty, non-faculty professional and support positions. Forty-eight percent are women and eight percent are minorities. Forty-seven percent are employed as faculty members, eight percent as executive, administrative and management, and eight percent as non-teaching professionals. The remaining 37% are employed as support staff. The subjects, who can participate in the program only once, were enrolled on a volunteer basis. A letter was mailed to each campus employee explaining the objectives of the program and inviting participation. Each year the program was limited to 30 participants. The first 30 to return the response form were enrolled. Once an employee had participated in the program, they were not eligible to participate again. The program requirements included participation in the knowledge and intervention components of the program, and completion of a pre-and post-program physiological assessment, and a blood lipid profile.

RESEARCH DESIGN

In order to test the first research hypothesis, the 154 subjects were collectively grouped and the data were analyzed to determine if a difference existed between the twelve component pre-and post-program physiological assessments. In order to test the remaining research hypotheses, the subjects were divided into two groups, pre-program exercisers and pre-program non-exercisers based on their answers to a set of interview questions. As part of the interview, the question was asked, "Have you engaged in a comprehensive fitness program three to five times per week at an intensity level of 60-80% of your age-adjusted maximal heart rate for a duration of 20 to 60 minutes for a minimum of one year prior to involvement in the wellness program?" Pre-program exercisers included subjects who affirmatively answered the preceding interview question. Pre-program non-exercisers included subjects who did not meet this threshold of activity for a minimum of one year prior to participation in the intervention program.

Within each group, subjects were sub-divided into those who increased exercise and those who did not increase exercise during the 16-week intervention program. This was determined by using a baseline of exercise as prescribed at the outset of the 16-week intervention program. The total number of aerobic minutes the participant exercised during the first four weeks of the intervention program were compared to the total number of aerobic minutes completed during the last four weeks. Subjects who increased total aerobic exercise time by $\geq 50\%$ were classified as subjects who increased exercise. Subjects classified as those who did not increase exercise included participants who did not meet this threshold of exercise increase during the 16-week intervention program. Therefore, the threshold of a $\geq 50\%$ increase in exercise time was used to differentiate the groups.

The research design for this study was quasi-experimental, as depicted below.

Group 1   11   XA 12
                 XB

Group 2   21   XA 22
                 XB

Group 1 included pre-program exercisers. Group 2 included pre-program non-exercisers. The first digit represents the group number, whereas, the second digit represents the assessment (i.e. 1=pre test, 2=post test). Therefore, the pre-test data were 11 and 21, and the post-test data were 12 and 22. XA represented participants who increased exercise ($\geq$50%), and XB represented participants who did not meet this threshold of exercise increase during the intervention program. Table 8.1 identifies descriptive characteristics of the groups and sub-groups used in this investigation.

RESEARCH VARIABLES

Two independent variables were included in this study. Each independent variable had two levels. The first independent variable was pre-program exercise level (categorized as either an exerciser, or a non-exerciser). The second independent variable was the extent of an increase in exercise time, quantified by an increase in total aerobic minutes (exercise duration) during the intervention program. This was calculated by comparing the total exercise time

TABLE 8.1 - Descriptive characteristics of the subjects participating in this investigation (groups and sub-groups)

Total Subjects: 154 Mean age: 39.2 ± 9.7 Females: 93 Males: 61				
	Group 1 Pre-program exercisers (N=68) mean age (37.8 ± 10.0) females=34 males=34		Group 2 Pre-program non-exercisers (N=86) mean age (40.2 ± 9.4) females=57 males=29	
	Increased exercise	Did not increase exercise	Increased exercise	Did not increase exercise
	N=28	N=40	N=36	N=50
females males	12 16	22 18	20 16	37 13

during the first four weeks as compared to the last four weeks of the intervention program. Two categories, or sub-groups were established. Subjects categorized as increasing exercise had to accomplish a $\geq 50\%$ increase in total exercise time. The subjects who failed to meet the established criterion were categorized as subjects who did not increase exercise. Twelve dependent variables were used to quantify the cardiovascular disease risk profile. The dependent variables included: (a) cardiovascular efficiency, systolic and diastolic blood pressure, estimated percent body fat, body mass index, and total body weight; (b) a lipid profile of total cholesterol, high density lipoproteins, low density lipoproteins, the ratio of total cholesterol to high density lipoproteins, and serum glucose.

TREATMENT OF THE DATA

In order to test the first research hypothesis, the groups were collapsed. In order to test the remaining research hypotheses, the subjects were grouped according to pre-program exercise level and the extent of an increase in total exercise time during the intervention program. While the total number of subjects included in this investigation was 154, the total number of subjects included in each analysis is dependent upon the number of matched pre- and post-test assessments for each dependent variable. LDL cholesterol could not be calculated for two subjects due to high (>400 mg/dl) triglyceride levels. Therefore, complete data sets per physiological variable were used in this investigation. A p value of .05 or less was considered significant in this investigation.

The first research hypothesis was tested using a dependent t-test and the second research hypothesis was tested using an independent t-test. These two hypotheses were:

1. There will be a significant difference (p<.05) in the cardiovascular disease risk profiles of subjects measured before and after participation in a 16-week health promotion program.

2. At entry, there will be a significant difference between the cardiovascular disease risk profiles of pre-program exercisers and pre-program non-exercisers.

The remaining research hypotheses (3-5) were tested using three separate multivariate analyses to test for a difference in the change scores of two groups.[11] These three hypotheses were:

3. There will be a significant difference between the cardiovascular disease risk profiles of subjects who increase exercise and subjects who do not increase exercise.
4. There will be a significant difference between the cardiovascular disease risk profiles of pre-program exercisers who increase exercise and pre-program exercisers who do not increase exercise.
5. There will be a significant difference between the cardiovascular disease risk profiles of pre-program non-exercisers who increase exercise and pre-program non-exercisers who do not increase exercise.

DATA ANALYSIS AND RESULTS

Remember, the purpose of this research was to investigate the effects of a 16-week university based health promotion program on cardiovascular disease risk profiles. A second objective was to investigate the specific influence of exercise on the cardiovascular disease risk profiles by assessing profile differences between active and non-active subjects at entry into the program, and by investigating how an increase in exercise duration affected the variables used to quantify the cardiovascular disease risk profile. Cardiovascular disease risk profiles were quantified through a comprehensive physiological assessment of cardiovascular fitness (estimated VO_2max), systolic and diastolic blood pressure, percent body fat, body mass index (BMI), weight and serum lipid levels of total cholesterol (TC), high density lipoproteins (HDL), low density lipoproteins (LDL), the ratio of TC to HDL, and the level of serum glucose. For the purpose of this investigation, complete data sets per physiological variable were used to quantify the cardiovascular disease risk profile. One hundred and fifty-four subjects participated in this investigation (mean age 39.2±9.7, range 25-60 years, females=93, males=61). The subjects were assessed and the physiological data collected prior to and after participation in a 16-week health promotion program. The purpose of this section is to present the data and discuss the results as they pertain to the research hypotheses for this study.

To review, the SRU Employee Wellness Program is a multi-faceted, educationally based health promotion program for the faculty and staff. The program consists of two components: knowledge and intervention. The knowledge component contains a multitude of services that are provided and available free of charge to all program participants. The standardized services include nutrition education and dietary analysis, and videotaped presentations on all aspects of health. The intervention component is comprised of an individualized wellness and exercise prescription that is based on the results of preliminary physiological and cognitive inventories. The exercise component of the intervention program follows the guidelines of the American College of Sports Medicine. Participants exercised three to five times per week for the duration of at least 20 minutes (up to 60 minutes) at a prescribed exercise intensity level of 60-80% of their age-adjusted maximal heart rate. Aerobic conditioning exercises were emphasized and were supplemented with resistance exercises; therefore, cardiovascular training preceded muscular strength and endurance conditioning.

The pre-program inventories consisted of a comprehensive physiological assessment, a three-day dietary analysis, and a five-component blood profile. The cognitive inventories consisted of a comprehensive health risk appraisal – The Lifestyle Assessment Questionnaire (5th edition LA-Q), and written information about each individual's medical history, exercise preferences, and program goals. After the 16 weeks, each participant was given a comprehensive post-program physiological assessment, and a detailed blood profile assessment.

THE CARDIOVASCULAR DISEASE RISK PROFILES OF SUBJECTS MEASURED BEFORE AND AFTER PARTICIPATION IN THE 16-WEEK HEALTH PROMOTION PROGRAM

Over the past 20 years, research studies have documented the efficacy of health promotion programs. A study by Health Promotion Services, a Blue Cross of Western Pennsylvania affiliate, reported a positive relationship between participation in a health promotion program, and health care utilization and cost control.[12] Chapman conducted an extensive analysis of the cost-effectiveness of employer sponsored health promotion programs and determined an average cost-benefit ratio of 1:5.94, with a range of 1:2.05 to 1:19.4.[13] Restated, for every dollar invested in an employee health promotion program, the average monetary return in savings was almost six dollars. Beyond the cost-effectiveness of health promotion programs, substantial research has suggested that the incidence of cardiovascular disease can be significantly reduced by an increase in physical activity.[14-18]

The relationship between an increase in physical activity and the reduction of chronic disease or conditions has also been examined. Blair conducted an in-depth analysis of studies investigating the benefits of physical activity on all-cause mortality, coronary artery disease, hypertension, obesity, and type 2 diabetes, and established excellent to good evidence of reduced disease rates.[19]

The first research hypothesis was tested in order to determine if a difference existed between the pre- and post-program physiological variables used to quantify the cardiovascular disease risk profile. A dependent t-test was used to test for a difference between the pre- and post-program mean value for each physiological variable. Table 8.2 presents the unadjusted means and standard deviations for the subjects prior to and after participation in the intervention program. The t ratios and the p values for the statistical analysis are also included. At entry, the mean value of 11 of the 12 variables fell within the recommended level for healthy adults. The mean value for total cholesterol, the variable that did not fall within the recommended range for healthy adults, was 202.05 mg/dl, which is only slightly above the recommended upper limit for healthy adults (200 mg/dl).

TABLE 8.2 - Group data prior to and after participation in the Employer Sponsored Health Promotion Intervention Program

Physiological Variable	N=	Pre-program value	Post-program value	t ratio	p ♦ value
CV-A (1/min)	110	2.30 ± .80	2.68 ± .83	6.49	.000*
CV-R(ml/kg/min)	110	31.26 ± 10.73	36.33 ± 10.69	6.74	.000*
SBP (mmHg)	131	119.83 ± 11.63	117.53 ± 11.23	2.98	.002*
DBP (mmHg)	131	76.63 ± 9.75	75.77 ± 9.66	1.15	.127
% body fat	128	26.61 ± 7.76	25.46 ± 7.18	3.04	.002*
BMI (kg/m^2)	129	26.11 ± 4.58	25.83 ± 4.29	3.13	.001*
Weight (lbs)	131	168.60 ± 34.95	166.86 ± 33.34	3.14	.001*
TC (mg/dl)	118	202.05 ± 38.50	196.90 ± 32.34	2.48	.007*
HDL (mg/dl)	116	50.54 ± 14.00	48.39 ± 13.90	3.15	>.050
LDL (mg/dl)	114	125.47 ± 34.99	122.46 ± 27.72	1.57	.060
TC:HDL	116	4.34 ± 1.52	4.43 ± 1.62	1.24	>.050
Glucose (mg/dl)	86	90.56 ± 9.82	91.71 ± 9.27	1.61	>.050

*p<.05   ♦ rounded to the third decimal

Statistically significant differences existed between pre- and post-program mean values for seven of the 12 cardiovascular disease risk variables. The most significant differences were evident in absolute (p=.000) and relative cardiovascular fitness (p=.000), BMI (p=.001), and body weight (p=.001). Systolic blood pressure (p=.002), percent body fat (p=.002), and total serum cholesterol (p=.007) were also significantly reduced. While not statistically significant, the mean value for low density lipoproteins (p=.060) and diastolic blood pressure (p=.127) dropped 2% and 1%, respectively. The direction of change in high density lipoproteins, the ratio of TC to HDL and glucose values was opposite of what was expected. It is postulated that HDL cholesterol may have slightly decreased due to the substantial decrease in total cholesterol, and consequentially also affected the ratio to TC to HDL cholesterol.

THE CARDIOVASCULAR DISEASE RISK PROFILES OF PRE-PROGRAM EXERCISERS AND PRE-PROGRAM NON-EXERCISERS AT ENTRY

Lower levels of habitual physical activity and cardiovascular fitness have been linked to coronary heart disease in strong and consistent epidemiological research, especially in middle-aged men.[20-21] Blair determined that adults in higher fitness categories have lower all-cause and cardiovascular disease mortality than those with the lowest fitness.[22] In a comprehensive review of the primary prevention effects of exercise, Powell concluded that more physically active people develop less CHD than their inactive counterparts.[18]

In order to determine whether physically active participants, at entry into the program, had different cardiovascular disease risk profiles compared to pre-program non-exercisers, the appropriate sub-groups were stratified. While self-reported information was used to differentiate the subgroups, an examination of the mean scores for each physiological variable and for each group revealed that the subjects had values indicative of relatively good cardiovascular health. Concurrently, the mean values appear to validate the subjects self-reported classification. An independent t-test was used to analyze the unadjusted means for the two groups. Table 8.3 presents the unadjusted means, standard deviations, t ratios, and the p values for the test of significance for pre-program exercisers and the pre-program non-exercisers prior to participation in the intervention program.

TABLE 8.3 - Group data for pre-program exercisers and pre-program non-exercisers at entry (same units as in Table 8.2)

Physiological Variable	N=	Pre-program exercisers	N=	Pre-program non-exercisers	t ratio	p ♦ value
CV-A	48	2.72 ± 0.83	62	1.97 ± 0.60	5.28	.000*
CV-R	48	38.01 ± 11.69	62	26.03 ± 6.08	6.46	.000*
SBP	62	118.82 ± 9.39	69	120.74 ± 13.33	0.96	.170
DBP	62	75.86 ± 8.51	69	77.32 ± 10.76	0.86	.200
% body fat	59	23.59 ± 7.77	69	29.19 ± 6.81	4.34	.000*
BMI	61	25.15 ± 4.07	68	26.96 ± 4.86	2.28	.012*
Weight	61	166.03 ± 34.86	70	170.83 ± 35.12	0.78	.217
TC	50	196.00 ± 36.23	68	206.50 ± 39.76	1.47	.070
HDL	50	51.62 ± 15.05	66	49.73 ± 13.22	0.72	.237
LDL	49	117.55 ± 33.59	65	131.45 ± 35.09	2.13	.020*
TC:HDL	50	4.15 ± 1.55	66	4.48 ± 1.48	1.16	.124
Glucose	37	89.00 ± 6.54	49	91.74 ± 11.64	1.38	.090

*p<.05   ♦ rounded to the third decimal

An examination of the mean values for the pre-program exercisers revealed that this group had numbers indicative of reduced cardiovascular disease risk in each of the 12 physiological variables used to quantify the cardiovascular disease risk profile. Statistically significant differences were found between the pre-program exercisers and non-exercisers in absolute (t=5.28, p=.000) and relative (t=6.46, p=.000) cardiovascular fitness, and percent body fat (t=4.34, p=.000). LDL cholesterol (t=2.13, p=.020), and BMI (t=2.28, p=.012) were also statistically different. While not statistically significant, total cholesterol values (t=1.47, p=.070) were 5.4% lower in the exercisers and the ratio of TC/HDL (t=1.16, p=.124) was 8% lower in the exercisers. The remaining variables were from 2-4% better in the exercisers.

It is important to note that with the exception of two variables, the pre-program non-exercising group mean values for cardiovascular disease risk factors fell within the recommended ranges for healthy adults. The two variables that did not fall within the recommended ranges included TC and LDL cholesterol. The recommended upper level for TC is <200 mg/dl, the pre-program non-exercising group mean value was 206 mg/dl. The recommended upper level for LDL cholesterol is <130 mg/dl, the subjects mean value was 131 mg/dl.

THE CARDIOVASCULAR DISEASE RISK PROFILES OF SUBJECTS WHO INCREASED EXERCISE AND SUBJECTS WHO DID NOT INCREASE EXERCISE

Epidemiological evidence has suggested that the incidence of cardiovascular disease can be significantly reduced by an increase in physical activity.[14-18] The physiological mechanisms have been thoroughly reviewed and explained earlier in this textbook, and have been described by Haskell who reported pathways whereby physical activity may contribute to the primary and secondary prevention of coronary artery disease.[23] The author describes an increase in myocardial oxygen supply, increased myocardial function, and decreased myocardial work and oxygen demand as all possible mechanisms leading to increased cardiovascular function.

Exercise has been shown to reduce serum cholesterol and to modify the lipid sub fractions that may also reduce cardiovascular risk.[24-26] As reported in observational studies, for each 1 mg/dl increase in HDL cholesterol, a corresponding reduction in CHD risk is approximately 2-3%. In clinical trials, a 1% reduction in total cholesterol has been associated with an average reduction in the incidence of CHD events by 2-3%. Research conducted by Gotto reported that a reduction in both total serum cholesterol and LDL cholesterol lowers the risk for CVD.[25]

In order to determine if a difference existed between people who increased exercise during the 16-week program and those who did not, the appropriate groups were stratified. A multivariate analysis to test for a difference in the change scores of two groups was used to analyze the data.[11] The unadjusted means, used to determine if a difference existed within the pre- and post-test data, standard deviations, F ratios, and p values are presented in Table 8.4.

TABLE 8.4 - Group data for subjects who increased exercise and subjects who did not increase exercise (same units as in Table 8.2)

Physiological Variable	N=	Subjects who increased exercise	N=	Subjects who did not increase exercise	F ratio	p ◆ value
Pre CV-A	57	2.25 ± 0.84	53	2.34 ± 0.76	33.8	.000*
Post CV-A		2.93 ± 0.92		2.35 ± 0.66		
Pre CV-R	57	30.25 ± 11.87	53	32.34 ± 9.35	38.7	.000*
Post CV-R		39.21 ± 12.28		33.23 ± 7.64		
Pre SBP	61	119.93 ± 11.37	70	119.74 ± 11.93	0.1	.748
Post SBP		117.36 ± 11.14		117.67 ± 11.38		
Pre DBP	61	77.46 ± 10.08	70	75.90 ± 9.46	0.9	.349
Post DBP		76.85 ± 9.56		75.70 ± 9.81		
Pre % fat	59	26.43 ± 8.28	69	26.77 ± 7.36	0.0	.927
Post % fat		25.23 ± 7.14		25.65 ± 7.26		
Pre BMI	61	26.62 ± 5.03	68	25.60 ± 4.12	4.4	.037*
Post BMI		25.23 ± 4.59		25.54 ± 4.02		
Pre weight	61	174.07 ± 37.90	70	163.83 ± 31.66	6.3	.014*
Post weight		170.87 ± 35.13		163.36 ± 31.53		
Pre TC	51	207.88 ± 40.23	67	197.61 ± 36.81	13.6	.000*
Post TC		194.39 ± 32.12		198.81 ± 32.63		
Pre HDL	50	48.90 ± 12.88	66	51.79 ± 14.77	5.4	.022*
Post HDL		48.54 ± 13.11		48.27 ± 14.56		
Pre LDL	50	131.82 ± 36.84	64	120.52 ± 32.92	12.3	.001*
Post LDL		121.54 ± 27.16		123.19 ± 28.34		
Pre TC:HDL	50	4.55 ± 1.49	66	4.17 ± 1.53	19.5	.000*
PostTC:HDL		4.30 ± 1.29		4.53 ± 1.83		
Pre glucose	35	92.20 ± 11.64	51	89.43 ± 8.29	8.3	.005*
Post glucose		90.97 ± 9.71		92.22 ± 9.01		˙

*p<.05   ◆ rounded to the third decimal

An examination of the data reveals that the subjects who were classified in the sub-group that increased exercise demonstrated significant differences in their change scores as compared to subjects who did not increase exercise. The most statistically significant differences were found within absolute (F=33.82, p=.000) and relative cardiovascular fitness (F=37.70, p=.000), total cholesterol (F=13.93, p=.000), and the ratio of TC/HDL (F=19.47, p=.000). Statistical significance was also reached in LDL cholesterol (F=12.30, p=.001), serum glucose (F=8.27, p=.005), body weight (F=6.25, p=.014), HDL cholesterol (F=5.41, p=.022), and BMI (F=4.42, p=.037).

THE CARDIOVASCULAR DISEASE RISK PROFILES OF PRE-PROGRAM EXERCISERS WHO INCREASED EXERCISE AND PRE-PROGRAM EXERCISERS WHO DID NOT INCREASE EXERCISE DURING THE INTERVENTION PROGRAM

Research has demonstrated that people who engage in regular fitness programs experience a reduction in cardiovascular disease risk. [17,19,27-28]

In order to determine the effects of the intervention program on pre-program exercisers who increased exercise, and pre-program exercisers who did not increase exercise, the appropriate groups were stratified and analyzed. A multivariate analysis to test for a difference in the change scores of two groups was used to analyze the data.[11] Table 8.5 presents the unadjusted means, standard deviations, F ratios, and p values when the group was subdivided into pre-program exercisers who increased exercise and pre-program exercisers who did not increase exercise.

Within the two groups, the most statistically significant differences were found in absolute (F=15.18, p=.000) and relative cardiovascular fitness (F=13.24, p=.001). LDL cholesterol (F=8.46, p=.006), total cholesterol (F=5.66, p=.021), and the ratio of TC/HDL cholesterol (F=5.24, p=.026) were also statistically different.

TABLE 8.5 - Group data for pre-program exercisers who increased exercise and pre-program exercisers who did not increase exercise during the intervention program (same units as in Table 8.2)

Physiological Variable	N=	Pre-program exercisers who increased exercise	N=	Pre-program exercisers who did not increase exercise	F ratio	p ♦ value
Pre CV-A	23	2.57 ± 0.93	25	2.86 ± 0.71	15.2	.000*
Post CV-A		3.24 ± 1.05		2.67 ± 0.77		
Pre CV-R	23	37.04 ± 14.42	25	38.90 ± 8.67	13.2	.001*
Post CV-R		45.37 ± 14.73		38.54 ± 6.83		
Pre SBP	26	117.58 ± 8.60	36	119.72 ± 9.94	1.2	.284
Post SBP		117.39 ± 11.11		117.19 ± 11.35		
Pre DBP	26	75.54 ± 8.81	36	76.08 ± 8.41	0.1	.826
Post DBP		74.62 ± 9.29		75.61 ± 8.76		
Pre % fat	25	22.91 ± 7.72	34	24.09 ± 7.88	2.0	.167
Post % fat		21.32 ± 6.64		23.68 ± 7.47		
Pre BMI	27	25.14 ± 4.82	34	25.17 ± 3.44	0.2	.623
Post BMI		24.90 ± 4.58		25.05 ± 3.49		
Pre weight	27	167.96 ± 40.35	34	164.50 ± 30.36	0.6	.428
Post weight		166.22 ± 37.92		163.94 ± 31.76		
Pre TC	23	201.91 ± 38.67	27	190.96 ± 33.93	5.7	.021*
Post TC		187.04 ± 32.22		190.37 ± 31.32		
Pre HDL	23	50.00 ± 15.97	27	53.00 ± 14.38	2.7	.106
Post HDL		49.83 ± 15.00		47.41 ± 11.81		
Pre LDL	23	124.13 ± 37.26	26	111.73 ± 29.48	8.5	.006*
Post LDL		113.83 ± 26.51		118.23 ± 28.26		
Pre TC:HDL	23	4.41 ± 1.63	27	3.93 ± 1.48	5.3	.026*
PostTC:HDL		4.07 ± 1.31		4.03 ± 1.31		
Pre glucose	15	88.80 ± 6.05	22	89.14 ± 6.99	2.4	.134
Post glucose		87.33 ± 7.89		90.91 ± 9.84		

*p<.05   ♦ rounded to the third decimal

Recent clinical studies support recommendations for exercise levels needed to reduce risk of cardiovascular disease. The American College of Sports Medicine and the Centers for Disease Control and Prevention recommend that Americans engage in moderate activity for at least 30 minutes most, preferably all, days of the week.[29] This level of activity should be sufficient to improve the physiological parameters related to cardiovascular disease risk. The exercise intervention of this investigation included participation in cardiovascular and strength conditioning exercises three to five times per week for a duration of 20 to 60 minutes at an intensity level of 60-80 % of the age-adjusted maximal heart rate. The threshold of activity required to be classified as increasing exercise was a ≥50% increase in exercise duration over the 16-week intervention program.

THE CARDIOVASCULAR DISEASE RISK PROFILES OF PRE-PROGRAM NON-EXERCISERS WHO INCREASED EXERCISE AND PRE-PROGRAM NON-EXERCISERS WHO DID NOT INCREASE EXERCISE DURING THE INTERVENTION PROGRAM

A major national health promotion and disease prevention objective for the current decade, as outlined in Healthy People 2000, and repeated in Healthy People 2010 is to increase physical activity levels among all Americans. Despite public health efforts, a large percentage of the population remains inactive. As reported in the 1996 Surgeon General's Report on Physical Activity and Health, more than 60% of American adults were not regularly physically active, and of that percentage, 25% were not active at all. In 2000, 40% of the population was inactive, and another 22% exercised less than they should.

Table 8.6 presents the unadjusted means, standard deviations, F ratios, and p values when the group was subdivided into pre-program non-exercisers who increased exercise and pre-program non-exercisers who did not increase exercise duration. A multivariate analysis to test for a difference in the change scores of the two groups was used to analyze the data.[11]

Within the pre- and post-test variables, the strongest significant differences in the change scores were evident in absolute and relative cardiovascular fitness (F=21.06, p=.000; F= 28.99 p=.000,

TABLE 8.6 - Group data for pre-program non-exercisers who increased exercise and pre-program non-exercisers who did not increase exercise during the intervention program (same units as in Table 8.2)

Physiological Variable	N=	Pre-program non-exercisers who increased exercise	N=	Pre-program non-exercisers who did not increase exercise	F ratio	p ♦ value
Pre CV-A	34	2.04 ± 0.71	28	1.87 ± 0.43	21.1	.000*
Post CV-A		2.72 ± 0.77		2.06 ± 0.36		
Pre CV-R	34	25.66 ± 6.83	28	26.48 ± 5.12	29.0	.000*
Post CV-R		35.05 ± 8.20		28.49 ± 4.62		
Pre SBP	35	121.69 ± 12.90	34	119.77 ± 13.89	1.5	.219
Post SBP		117.34 ± 11.33		118.18 ± 11.55		
Pre DBP	35	78.89 ± 10.84	34	75.71 ± 10.58	1.0	.321
Post DBP		76.77 ± 9.80		75.79 ± 10.95		
Pre % fat	34	29.01 ± 7.80	35	29.37 ± 5.81	0.56	.457
Post % fat		28.11 ± 6.11		27.56 ± 6.60		
Pre BMI	34	27.80 ± 4.94	34	26.12 ± 4.70	4.9	.030*
Post BMI		27.13 ± 4.41		26.04 ± 4.48		
Pre weight	34	178.91 ± 35.69	36	163.19 ± 33.26	6.3	.014*
Post weight		174.56 ± 32.85		162.81 ± 32.21		
Pre TC	28	212.79 ± 41.52	40	202.10 ± 38.39	7.5	.008*
Post TC		200.43 ± 31.31		204.50 ± 32.63		
Pre HDL	27	47.96 ± 9.75	39	50.95 ± 15.16	2.6	.111
Post HDL		47.44 ± 11.45		47.49 ± 16.30		
Pre LDL	27	138.37 ± 35.86	38	126.53 ± 34.15	4.6	.036*
Post LDL		128.11 ± 27.23		126.58 ± 28.47		
Pre TC:HDL	27	4.67 ± 1.38	39	4.34 ± 1.56	14.2	.000*
PostTC:HDL		4.49 ± 1.27		4.87 ± 2.06		
Pre glucose	20	94.75 ± 14.13	29	89.66 ± 9.27	6.0	.018*
Post glucose		93.70 ± 10.23		93.21 ± 8.37		

*p<.05   ♦ rounded to the third decimal

respectively), and the ratio of TC/HDL cholesterol (F=14.18, p=.000). Total cholesterol (F=7.53, p=.008), body weight (F=6.34, p=.014), serum glucose (F=5.99, p=.018), BMI (F=4.91, p=.030), and LDL cholesterol (F=4.58, p=.036) were also significantly different. Between the pre-program non-exercisers who increased exercise and the pre-program non-exercisers who did not increase exercise, a statistical significant difference was reached in 8 of the 12 change scores. This sub group analysis demonstrated significant improvements and dramatic results in a majority of the variables measured and used to quantify the cardiovascular disease risk profile. Public health officials have long contented that a small increase in activity among the least active segment of our population could dramatically improve health and decrease cardiovascular disease risk factors, subsequently lowering cardiovascular disease rates. This data supports these assumptions, and supports the need to focus public health efforts towards the least active segments of our population.

DISCUSSION OF THE RESULTS

The following discussion focuses on the effects of the intervention program on the physiological variables used to quantify the cardiovascular disease risk profile. The section has been divided into four categories: 1) cardiovascular fitness; 2) percent body fat, BMI and body weight; 3) blood pressure and, 4) blood lipids and serum glucose.

CARDIOVASCULAR FITNESS

The effects of this employer sponsored health promotion program on the variables used to assess cardiovascular fitness are consistent with studies that qualified an increase in VO_2 max. in response to participation in an exercise program.[30-33] In comparing the pre to post test assessments (Table 8.2), the participants in this study experienced a mean increase of 17% in the estimated VO_2 max when training was accompanied with changes in body composition. Percent body fat, BMI, and weight decreased in this study, which may have precipitated an additional increase in VO_2 max. It is comparable to research completed by Wilmore reported an average increase in VO_2 max of 15-20% in sedentary persons following participation in an exercise program consisting of three times per week for 30 minutes at 75% of capacity and research that has found an increase in VO_2 max of between 5-30%.[30-31,33] The 16-week intervention program was effective at improving cardiovascular fitness values, as both pre program exercisers and pre program non-exercises experienced substantial improvements. While pre program exercisers improved 26%, pre program non-exercisers improved 33%. This finding is consistent with the literature that has demonstrated greater improvements in less active subjects. Habitual exercisers, as compared to non-exercisers (Table 8.3), had statistically significantly higher absolute and relative cardiovascular fitness values and when comparing absolute cardiovascular fitness values, the habitual exercisers were 38% higher. The results of the group and sub-group analyses demonstrated the effectiveness of the intervention program on cardiovascular fitness, as in each analysis, the improvements were statistically significant at $p<0.01$. This research supports a study in which Finnish investigators reported a strong, graded, inverse association between physical inactivity and cardiovascular fitness.[34]

PERCENT BODY FAT, BMI, AND BODY WEIGHT

Research studies on the effects of health promotion programs on BMI, weight, and percent body fat have indicated a possible synergistic effect of nutrition intervention and exercise on improved values.[24,35-37] As part of this program, nutrition information was combined with exercise intervention. In this investigation, a combination of exercise and nutritional intervention may have led to the significant improvements in the body fat, BMI, and body weight.

Physical activity has been shown to modify cardiovascular disease risk factors such as obesity and undesirable blood lipid profiles.[38] The National Institutes of Health consensus statement has defined obesity as an excess of body fat frequently resulting in a significant impairment of health. Research studies have demonstrated that obesity is associated with reduced longevity and increased incidence of cardiovascular disease and diabetes mellitus.[39-40] In an in-depth analysis, researchers determined that physical activity affects body composition favorably by promoting fat loss while preserving lean mass.[41] The investigation also found a clear dose-response relationship between those who exercised longer and more often, and an increased rate of weight loss.

In this investigation, percent body fat, BMI, and body weight were significantly reduced after participation in the intervention program (Table 8.2). At entry, BMI was 7% lower in the habitual exercisers (Table 8.3). This study confirms previous research that physically active individuals have lower body fat, BMI, body weight, and improved lipid profiles. Subjects who increased aerobic exercise ($\geq$50%), in this investigation, (Table 8.4) experienced a significant reduction in BMI and body weight; however, percent body fat was not significantly different between subjects who increased aerobic exercise ($\geq$50%) and subjects who did not increase exercise. In the subgroup analyses (Tables 8.5 and 8.6), there were no significant differences in the change scores in percent body fat, BMI or body weight in the pre-program exercisers who increased exercise as compared to the pre-program exercisers who did not increase exercise. In the pre-program non-exercisers, BMI and body weight were significantly different; however, the change score for percent body fat was not significantly different regardless of the change in aerobic exercise participation. The changes may have been greater had the mean value for these variables not fallen within the recommended range for healthy adults.

BLOOD PRESSURE

Hypertension is associated with higher cardiovascular morbidity and morality rates and is prevalent in 28% of adults in the U.S. (age-adjusted to the year 2000 standard population).[6] While the subjects in this investigation experienced a 2.3 mmHg reduction in systolic blood pressure, other researchers determined an average reduction in systolic blood pressure of between 6-10 mmHg with regular aerobic exercise.[32] The difference may be attributed to the fact that the subjects in this investigation, at entry, had relatively good blood pressure values. The reduction in SBP after participation in the intervention program (Table 8.2) was significant; however, the reduction in DBP was not significant. This study is consistent with research that has shown that active individuals have lower SBP and DBP readings than inactive adults.[32-33,42] While the mean values for the subjects did drop after participation in the program, there were no significant differences between subjects who increased aerobic exercise and subjects who did not increase aerobic exercise (Table 8.4), or in the subgroup analyses for both SBP and DBP (Tables 8.5 and 8.6). The largest improvements in the mean values, for both SBP and DBP, were evident in pre-program non-exercisers who increased exercise. It is important to note that the baseline values for SBP and DBP fell within the recommended range. Therefore, the mean changes for both SBP and DBP were greatest in those subjects who were most sedentary at entry but increased aerobic exercise $\geq 50\%$ during the intervention program.

BLOOD LIPIDS AND FASTING SERUM GLUCOSE

In this investigation, pre-program exercisers, as compared to pre-program non-exercisers, had a higher mean value of HDL cholesterol and a lower mean value of LDL cholesterol (Table 8.3). This finding is consistent with previously published research that found higher HDL and lower LDL cholesterol levels in physically active versus inactive adults.[43] The mean values for total cholesterol, HDL cholesterol, and the ratio of TC/HDL cholesterol, while not significantly different, were better in the participants who were habitual exercisers. The difference in LDL cholesterol was significantly different between habitual exercisers and non-exercisers and was 12% lower in the habitual exercisers.

In comparing the mean values for all subjects prior to and after participation in the intervention program (Table 8.2), total cholesterol significantly dropped. Non-significant directional changes were evident in the lipid sub-fractions as LDL and HDL cholesterol decreased and the corresponding ratio of TC/HDL cholesterol increased.

While the documented reduction in total serum cholesterol has been supported by research,[44-45] inconsistent findings have been reported for changes in lipoprotein sub-fractions as a result of exercise intervention programs.[44-47] Some researchers believe this may be related to a lack of control in the experimental variables.[48-49] While specific research[26] supports a possible gender related difference in the variation in HDL cholesterol following exercise, collateral research[50] found HDL increases only when exercise is combined with a corresponding loss of weight. There appears to be a general consensus that a combination of exercise and weight loss contributes to a change in the lipid subfractions.[26,51] However, in this investigation, a corresponding weight loss and decreases in BMI and percent body fat accompanied reductions in total cholesterol and LDL cholesterol, but HDL cholesterol also decreased.

Kris-Etherton found that exercise decreases total cholesterol sometimes in certain studies and in other studies there in no change in total cholesterol.[26] This may be related less to changes in the level of total cholesterol and more to changes in the lipid sub-fractions, possibly related to a combination of changes in other physiological variables. Haskell and Bryant suggest the modification of the enzymes involved in triglyceride and cholesterol synthesis, transport, and catabolism may mediate the changes in lipid sub-fractions resulting from exercise.[45,52] According to Hurley and Bouchard, the relationship between exercise and the lipid sub-fractions appears variable and inconclusive.[53-54]

While there appears to be a lack of consensus in the literature regarding the effects of exercise on the lipid sub-fractions, further data analyses of the subgroup of subjects who increased exercise duration ($\geq$ 50%) are revealing. The intervention program appears to have had the greatest effect on the blood lipids in those subjects who increased exercise duration ($\geq$50%), regardless of pre-program exercise level. Within the subgroup analyses, total cholesterol, LDL cholesterol, and the ratio of TC/HDL cholesterol were statistically significantly different between subjects who increased exercise duration ($\geq$50%), and subjects who did not increase exercise duration. This was a consistent finding in both the pre-program exercisers and the pre-program non-exercisers.

The variability within the lipid sub-fractions is limited to HDL cholesterol, which fell within each group and subgroup analyses. The reductions were consistently greater, although statistically non-significantly different, in those subjects who did not increase exercise duration. The consistent decreases in HDL cholesterol may have been related to a combination of relatively healthy HDL cholesterol at entry into the program, and concomitant changes in other measured physiological variables.

The changes in fasting serum glucose were not significantly different between the pre- and post-test assessment, between pre-program exercisers as compared to pre-program non-exercisers, or between pre-program exercises who increased exercise and pre-program exercisers who did not increase exercise. The difference in the change scores were statistically significantly different between subjects who increased exercise and subjects who did not increase exercise, and between pre-program non-exercisers who increased exercise and pre-program non-exercisers who did not increase exercise. The mean level of fasting serum glucose, across all group and subgroup stratifications, fell within the recommended range for healthy adults. This fact may help explain less dramatic changes in fasting serum glucose for subjects in this study.

SUMMARY

Remember, the purpose of this chapter was to thoroughly investigate the physiological effects of a 16-week university based health promotion program on cardiovascular disease risk profiles, and to document physiological efficacy. A second objective was to investigate the specific influence of exercise on the cardiovascular disease risk profiles by assessing profile differences between active and non-active subjects at entry into the program, and by investigating how an increase in exercise duration affected the variables used to quantify the cardiovascular disease risk profile. Cardiovascular disease risk profiles were quantified through a comprehensive physiological assessment of cardiovascular fitness, systolic and diastolic blood pressure, percent body fat, body mass index (BMI), weight, and serum lipid levels of total cholesterol (TC), high density lipoproteins (HDL), low density lipoproteins (LDL), the ratio of TC to HDL, and the level of serum glucose. This study included data taken from the physiological assessments of the subjects who participated in an employee based health promotion program at Slippery Rock University. Complete data sets per physiological variable were used to quantify the cardiovascular disease risk profile.

One hundred and fifty four subjects participated in this study (mean age 39.2 ± 9.7, range 25-60 years, females=93, males= 61). Subjects were divided into two groups, pre-program exercisers and pre-program non-exercisers based on their answers to a set of interview questions. Pre-program exercisers included people who had participated in a comprehensive fitness program three to five times per week at an intensity level of 60-80% of their age-adjusted maximal heart rate for the duration of 20 to 60 minutes for a minimum of one year prior to involvement in the intervention program. Pre-program non-exercisers were people who did not meet this threshold of activity for a minimum of one year prior to participation in the program. Within each group, the subjects were subdivided into those who increased exercise duration and those who did not increase exercise during the 16-week intervention program. Subjects who increased exercise experienced a ≥50% increase in total aerobic exercise time during the intervention program. This was determined by using a baseline of exercise as prescribed at the outset of the 16-week intervention program. The total number of aerobic minutes the participant exercised during the first four weeks of the intervention program were compared to the total number of aerobic minutes completed during the last four weeks of the intervention program. Subjects who increased total aerobic exercise time by $\geq 50\%$ were classified as subjects who increased exercise. Subjects classified as those who did not increase exercise did not meet this threshold of increase during the 16-week intervention program.

The purpose of this section is to summarize the research findings, provide conclusions based upon the research findings, and provide recommendations for further research.

The following research findings were identified in this investigation.

1. Based upon the pre- and post-program physiological assessments, which were taken before and after participation in a 16-week employee based health promotion program, the subjects experienced significant improvements ($p<0.05$) in seven of the twelve variables used to quantify the cardiovascular disease risk profile. The seven variables included absolute ($p=.000$) and relative ($p=.000$) cardiovascular fitness, BMI ($p=.001$), weight ($p=.001$), systolic blood pressure ($p=.002$), percent body fat ($p=.002$), and total cholesterol ($p=.007$). The mean value of two of the twelve variables improved, but did not reach statistical significance, diastolic blood pressure ($p=.127$) and low density lipoproteins ($p=.060$). The mean value of three variables moved in an opposite direction relative to cardiovascular disease risk. These variables included high density lipoproteins, the ratio of TC to HDL, and serum glucose.

2. At entry, pre-program exercisers as compared to pre-program non-exercisers had cardiovascular disease risk profiles indicative of reduced cardiovascular disease risk on each of the 12 physiological variables. Statistically significant differences were found in absolute ($p=.000$) relative ($p=.000$) cardiovascular fitness, percent body fat ($p=.000$), body mass index ($p=0.12$), and low

density lipoproteins (p=.020). Pre-program exercisers, as compared to non-exercisers had 5.4% lower total cholesterol, and the ratio of TC/HDL was 8% lower. The remaining variables were from 2-4% better in the exercisers.

3. Subjects who increased exercise duration demonstrated improved cardiovascular disease risk profiles. Statistically significantly differences in the change scores between subjects who increased exercise and subjects who did not increase exercise were found within absolute (p=.000) and relative (p=.000) cardiovascular fitness, total cholesterol (p=.000), and the ratio TC to HDL cholesterol (p=.000). LDL cholesterol (p=.001), serum glucose (p=.005), body weight (p=.014), HDL cholesterol (p=.022), and BMI (p=.037) were also significantly different. The differences in the change scores for systolic and diastolic blood pressure and percent body fat were not significantly different.

4. Pre-program exercisers who increased exercise duration experienced improved cardiovascular disease risk profiles. Statistically significant differences in the change scores between pre-program exercisers who increased exercise and pre-program exercisers who did not increase exercise were found within absolute (p=.000) and relative (p=.001) cardiovascular fitness. LDL cholesterol (p=.006), total cholesterol (p=.021), and the ratio of TC/HDL cholesterol (p=.026) were also significantly different.

5. Pre-program exercisers who increased exercise duration experienced improvements in the quantified cardiovascular disease risk profile. Statistically significant differences in the change scores between the pre-program exercisers who increased exercise and pre-program exercisers who did not increase exercise were found within absolute (p=.000) and relative (p=.000) cardiovascular fitness, and the ratio of TC/HDL cholesterol (p=.000). Significant differences in the change scores were also evident in total cholesterol (p=.008), body weight (p=.014), serum glucose (p=.018), BMI (p=.030), and LDL cholesterol (p=.036).

CONCLUSIONS

Within the limitations of this investigation, the aforementioned results support the following conclusions.

1. Subjects who participated in this investigation experienced statistically significant ($p \leq .05$) improvements in seven of the twelve physiological variables used to quantify the cardiovascular disease risk profile. The largest improvements throughout the 16-week interventions program were evident in absolute and relative cardiovascular fitness ($p \leq .001$).

2. Subjects who achieved a $\geq 50\%$ increase in aerobic exercise duration, as compared to subjects who did increase aerobic exercise duration, across all group and sub-group analyses, experienced a statistically significantly reduction in TC, LDL cholesterol, and the ratio of TC to HDL cholesterol. The mean value of HDL cholesterol decreased in each group, regardless of exercise participation level. Participants who did not increase exercise duration $\geq 50\%$ during the intervention program, experienced slight mixed directional changes in the physiological variables used to quantify the cardiovascular disease risk profile.

3. The mean value for the level of serum glucose was significantly different in the subjects who increased exercise ($\geq 50\%$) as compared to the subjects who did not increase exercise, and within the pre-program non-exercisers who increased exercise as compared to the pre-program non-exercisers who did not increase exercise. The change in the level of serum glucose was not significantly different in the pre-program exercisers who increased exercise as compared to the pre-program exercisers who did not increase exercise.

4. The mean value of percent body fat, BMI, and body weight dropped in all groups and sub-groups throughout the

intervention program. The change in BMI and body weight were statistically different ($p \leq .05$) in the subjects who increased exercise as compared to the subjects who did not increase exercise, and in the pre-program non-exercisers who increased exercise as compared to the pre-program non-exercisers who did not increase. The difference in the change score was not significantly different in the pre-program exercisers who increased exercise as compared to the pre-program exercisers who did not increase exercise.

Percent body fat was not significantly different in the sub-groups that increased exercise as compared to the sub-groups that did not increase exercise. BMI, body weight, and serum glucose were significantly different in the subjects who increased exercise, and in the pre-program non-exercisers who increased exercise, but not significantly different in the pre-program exercisers who increased exercise.

5. The mean value for systolic blood pressure and percent body fat, while statistically different before as compared to after the intervention program, were not significantly different ($p \leq .05$) within each group and sub-group analysis.

6. LDL cholesterol and the ratio of TC to HDL cholesterol, while not significantly different ($p \leq .05$) before as compared to after the intervention program, reached statistical significance within each group and sub-group analysis.

7. In comparing the subjects who increased exercise ($\geq 50\%$) and the subjects who did not increase exercise during the intervention program, statistical significance ($p \leq .05$) was evident in the change scores of nine of the twelve variables. Within the pre-programs exercisers, five of the twelve variables were significantly different and within the pre-program non-exercisers, eight of the twelve variables were significantly different.

RECOMMENDATIONS FOR FURTHER RESEARCH

Based upon the research findings and conclusions, the following recommendations are suggested for further research.

1.   A longer intervention program (i.e. six months rather than 16 weeks) should be investigated to determine if length of the study was a factor in eliciting specific physiological results.

2.   At entry, the mean value of 11 of the 12 variables used to quantify the cardiovascular disease risk profile fell within the recommended ranges. This investigation should be replicated with subjects who have physiological values indicative of increased cardiovascular disease risk.

3.   This research study used a $\geq 50\%$ increase in total aerobic exercise time to classify subjects as experiencing an increase in exercise. Since exercise intensity has been reported to be a variable that may affect physiological changes related to cardiovascular health, the study should be replicated incorporating a measurement of exercise intensity.

4.   For comparative purposes, this study should be replicated with a control group.

5.   Since a major objective of the health promotion program is to affect long-term behavioral change, a follow-up investigation should be initiated in order to document long-term adherence.

REFERENCES

1.   Opatz, J.P. (1986). "Stevens Point: A longstanding program for students at a midwestern university." *American Journal of Health Promotion* 1, 60-67.

2. McMillan, L. (1986). "Colleges finding wellness programs cut absenteeism, boost productivity and morale of their staff members." *The Chronicles of Higher Education* 31(23), 20-22.

3. U.S. Department of Health and Human Services. (1993). "1992 national survey of worksite health promotion activities: Summary." *American Journal of Health Promotion* 7, 264-452.

4. Caler, C.A. (1996). "University health promotion programs in the Pennsylvania State System of Higher Education." Unpublished master's thesis, The Pennsylvania State University, State College, Pennsylvania.

5. U.S. Department of Health and Human Services. (1990). *Healthy People 2000 National Health Promotion and Disease Prevention Objectives.* (DHHS Publication No PHS 91-50213). Washington, DC: Government Printing Office (5)392-395.

6. Neiman, D.C. (2003). *Exercise Testing and Prescription a Health Related Approach.* (pp. 80-84, 130, 385). New York, NY: McGraw-Hill Higher Education.

7. Golding, L.A., Myers, C.R., & Sinning, W.E. (Eds.). (1989). *Y's Way to Physical Fitness: The Complete Guide to Fitness Testing and Instruction.* (3rd ed., pp. 89-106). Champaign: Human Kinetics.

8. Ng, N.K. (1995). *METCALC Software: Metabolic Calculations in Exercise and Fitness.* Champaign: Human Kinetics.

9. Allain, C.C., Poon, L.S., Chan, C.S.G., Richmond, W., & Fu, P.C. (1974). *Clinical Chemistry* 20, 470-475.

10. Slein, M.W. (1963). *D-Glucose: Determination with Hexokinase and Glucose 6-Phosphate Dehydrogenase Methods of Enzymatic Analysis.* New York: Academic Press.

11. Bruning, J., & Kintz, B. (1997). *Computational Handbook of Statistics*. New York: Longman.

12. Papale, M.A. & Lawless, G.D. (1993). "The impact of lifestyle health risk on the bottom line: A case study." *Employee Benefits Journal* 18, 19-21.

13. Chapman, L.S. (1995). "Meta-Analysis of Studies on the Cost-Effectiveness of Worksite Health Promotion Programs." Paper presented at the meeting of the American Journal of Health Promotion, Orlando, FL.

14. Blair, S. (1996). "Physical inactivity and cardiovascular disease risk in women." *Medicine and Science in Sports and Exercise* 28, 9-10.

15. Blair, S. (1994). "Physical activity, fitness, and coronary heart disease." In C. Bouchard, R.J. Shepard, & T. Stephens (Eds.), *Physical Activity, Fitness, and Health: International Proceedings and Consensus Statement.* (pp. 579-590). Champaign: Human Kinetics.

16. Blair, S. & McCloy, C.H. (1993). "Research lecture: physical activity, physical fitness, and health." *Research Quarterly in Exercise* 64, 365-376.

17. Paffenberger, R.S., Hyde, R.T., Wing, A.L., Lee, I.M., Jung, D.L., & Kampert, J.B. (1993). "The association of changes in physical activity level and other lifestyle characteristics with mortality among men." *New England Journal of Medicine* 328, 538-545.

18. Powell, K.E., Thompson, P.D., Casperton, C., & Kendrick, J.S. (1987). "Physical activity and the incidence of coronary heart disease." *American Review of Public Health* 8, 253-287.

19. Blair, S. (1995). "Effects of physical activity on cardiovascular disease mortality independent of risk factors: Physical Activity and Cardiovascular Health." NIH Consensus Development Conference Abstract, 77-83.

20. Berlin, J.A., & Colditz, G.A. (1990). "A meta-analysis of physical activity in the prevention of coronary heart disease." *American Journal of Epidemiology* 132, 612-628.

21. Centers for Disease Control and Prevention. (1993). "Public health focus: Physical activity and the prevention of coronary heart disease." *Morbidity Mortality Weekly Report* 42, 669-672.

22. Blair, S.N., Kohl III, H.W., Paffenberger, R.S., Clark, G.G., Cooper, K.H., & Gibbons, L.W. (1989). "Physical fitness and all-cause mortality." *Journal of the American Medical Association* 262, 2395-2401.

23. Haskell, W.L. (1994). "Sedentary lifestyle as a risk factor for coronary heart disease." In T.A. Pearson, M.H. Criqui, R.K. Luepker, A. Oberman, & M. Winston (Eds.), *AHA Primer in Preventive Cardiology.* (pp. 173-188). Dallas: American Heart Association.

24. Cooper, E.S., & Lenfant, C.M. (1993). *Exercise and Your Heart: A Guide to Physical Activity.* Dallas: American Heart Association.

25. Gotto, A.M. (1994). "Lipid and lipoprotein disorders." In T.A. Pearson, M.H. Criqui, R.K. Luepker, A. Oberman, & M. Winston (Eds.), *AHA Primer in Preventive Cardiology.* (pp. 107-129). Dallas: American Heart Association.

26. Kris-Etherton, P.M. (1990). *Cardiovascular Disease: Nutrition for Prevention and Treatment.* (pp. 24-25). Chicago: The American Dietetic Association.

27. Blair, S.N., Kohl III, H.W., & Gordon, N.F. (1992). "Physical activity and health: A lifestyle approach." *Medicine in Exercise, Nutrition, and Health* 1, 54-7.

28. Caspersen, C.J., Powell, K.E., & Christenson, G.M. (1987). "Physical activity and coronary heart disease." *The Physician and Sports Medicine* 15, 43-44.

29. Pate, R.R., et al. (1995). "Physical activity and public health: A recommendation from the center for disease control and prevention and the American College of Sports Medicine." *Journal of the American Medical Association* 273, 402-407.

30. American College of Sports Medicine. (1995). *Guidelines for Exercise Testing and Prescription*. (5th ed., p. 156). Baltimore: Williams and Wilkins.

31. Booth, F.W., & Thompson, D.B. (1991). "Molecular and cellular adaptation of muscle in response to exercise: Perspectives of various models." *Physiological Reviews* 71, 547-559, 566-573.

32. McArdle, W.D., Katch, F.I., & Katch, V.L. (2001). *Exercise Physiology: Energy, Nutrition, and Human Performance*. (5th ed., pp. 468-485). Boston: Williams and Wilkins.

33. Wilmore, J.H., & Costill, D.L. (1994). *Physiology of Sport and Exercise*. (pp. 222-239). Champaign: Human Kinetics.

34. Lakka, T.A., Venalainen, J.M., Rauramaa, R., Salonen, R., Tuomilehto, J., & Salonen, J.T. (1994). "Relation of leisure-time physical activity and cardiorespiratory fitness to the risk of acute myocardial infarction." *New England Journal of Medicine* 330, 1549-1554.

35. Aldana, S.G., Jacobson, B.H., & Kelley, P.L. (1993). "Mobile work site health promotion program can reduce selected employee health risks." *Journal of Occupational Medicine* 35, 922-928.

36. Briley, M.E., Montgomery, D.W., & Blewett, J. (1992). "Worksite nutrition education can lower total cholesterol levels and promote weight loss among police department employees." *Journal of the American Dietetic Association* 92, 1372-1384.

37. Hellenius, M.L., DeFaire, U., Bergkard, B., Hamster, A:, & Krakau, I. (1993). "Diet and exercise are equally effective in controller study in men with slightly to moderately raised cardiovascular risk factors." *Atherosclerosis* 103, 81-91.

38. Bouchard, C., Shephard, R.J., & Stephens, T. (Eds.). (1994). *Physical Activity, Fitness, and Health.* Champaign: Human Kinetics.

39. National Institutes of Health Consensus Panel. (1985). "Health implications of obesity: NIH Consensus Development Conference Statement." *Annals of Internal Medicine* 103, 1073-1077.

40. National Research Council. (1989). "Diet and health: Implications for reducing chronic disease." Washington, DC: National Academy Press.

41. DiPietro, L. (1995). "Physical activity, body weight, and adiposity: An epidemiologic perspective." *Exercise and Sport Science Reviews* 27, 281-296.

42. Hagberg, J.M. (1995). "Physical activity, physical fitness, and blood pressure." NIH Consensus Development Conference Abstract, 69-71.

43. Stefanick, M.L. (1995). "Physical activity and lipid metabolism." NIH Consensus Development Conference Abstract, 65-67.

44. Goldberg, L., Elliot, D.L, & Schultz, R.W. (1984). "Changes in lipid lipoprotein levels after weight training." *Journal of the American Medical Association* 225, 504.

45. Haskell, W.L. (1984). "Exercise-induced changes in plasma lipids and lipoproteins." *Preventative Medicine* 13, 23.

46. Cook, T.C., Laprote, R.E., & Washburn, R.A. (1986). "Chronic low level physical activity as a determinant of high density lipoprotein cholesterol and subfractions." *Medicine and Science in Sports and Exercise* 18, 653.

47. Frey, M.A.B., Doerr, B.M., & Laubach, L.L. (1982). "Exercise does not change high-density lipoprotein cholesterol in women after ten weeks of training." *Metabolism* 31, 1142.

48. McManus, B.M. (1985). "Defining coronary risks in a reference range for total cholesterol and lipoprotein values: A problem yet to be solved." *American Journal of Cardiology* 13, 1-3.

49. Miettinen, T.A. (1985). "Multifactorial primary prevention of cardiovascular disease in middle-aged men." *Journal of the American Medical Association* 254, 2097-2102.

50. Hamilton, E.N., Whitney, E.N., & Sizer, F.S. (1991). *Nutrition Concepts and Controversies.* (5th ed., pp. 134-135). St. Paul: West.

51. McCunney, R.J. (1987). "Fitness, heart disease, and high-density lipoproteins: a look at the relationships." *The Physician and Sportsmedicine* 15, 67-76.

52. Bryant, S. (1990). "Exercise intervention for CHD. Cardiovascular Disease: Nutrition for prevention and treatment." *Journal of the American Dietetic Association* 90, 192-224.

53. Hurley, B.F., Seals, D.R., & Hagberg, J.M. (1984). "High-density-lipoprotein cholesterol in bodybuilders versus powerlifters: Negative effects of androgen use." *Journal of the American Medical Association* 254, 507.

54. Bouchard, C. (1995). "Overview of the biological and physiological mechanisms by which different forms of physical activity prevent cardiovascular disease." NIH Consensus Development Conference Abstract, 37-40.

CHAPTER NINE

SUMMARY AND CONCLUSIONS

This chapter reviews, highlights, and summarizes the previous chapters.

Chronic disease accounts for approximately 75% of health care costs each year.[1] The number one contributor to health care costs and the leading chronic disease contributor to premature morbidity and mortality in the nation is cardiovascular disease (CVD).[2] In 1990, the estimated cost of CVD was $135 billion.[3] In 2003, it is expected to reach $209 billion, a 55% increase.[1] Epidemiological evidence has suggested that the incidence of cardiovascular disease can be significantly reduced by an increase in physical activity.[4-7] Research studies have demonstrated that a sedentary person runs almost twice the risk of developing heart disease than the most active person.[7] Substantial epidemiological evidence has suggested that employee sponsored health promotion programs can improve the risk factors for cardiovascular disease and reduce the ever increasing burden of health care costs.

The escalating cost of health care is slowly outpacing society's ability to pay for it. In 1960, national health expenditures consumed

5.1% of the Gross Domestic Product (GDP) or $27 billion. In 1985, the numbers grew to 10.1 % of the GDP, or $430 billion. In the year 2003, the cost rose to 15.2% of the GDP, as Americans spent $1.66 trillion on Health Care. Government projections estimate that health care costs will increase about 7% annually though the next decade as the cost of hospital services and prescription drugs continue to increase. Projections for health care expenditures from 2008-2012 predict that consumers will spend $2.4 trillion in 2008, $3 trillion in 2010, and $3.1 trillion, or 17.7% of the GDP by 2012, and an astonishing $13 trillion, or 26% of GNP, by 2030.[8-9] With an average expenditure of about $5,000.00 per citizen, Americans spend more money on health care than any other country in the world.[1]

A comprehensive review, published in 1999, analyzed return on investment (ROI) data from studies on corporate health and productivity management initiatives.[10] The results of this investigation indicate a broad range of return on investment estimates and calculations. This range spanned from a low of $1.49 in benefits per dollar spent to a high of $13. The range was dependent on the type of program offered, and the available data used for analysis. Nine studies were included in the analysis on corporate health management ROIs. The range of benefit-to-cost ratios for these programs was about $1.50-$4.90 in benefits per dollar spent on the program. The median ROI was about $3.14 in benefits per dollar spent. Study participants included in the research analyses investigated ranged from 517 to 49,249.

Perhaps more important than the cost-efficacy of preventive programs is the shift in the emphasis of health promotion programs from a focus on productivity to an improvement of health, with more altruistic companies viewing this as a beneficial social goal in itself. Initial research studies on the physiological benefits of employer sponsored health promotion programs have provided a foundation to build the argument for the appropriation of resources for preventive programs.

A plethora of health promotion programs were researched, reviewed, and analyzed. A cross-section of public, private, large and small, from throughout the country were included for reference. Detailed information was provided on program components, employee demographics, and evaluation efforts.

The detailed analysis of the selected university based health promotion program provided evidence of physiological efficacy on twelve variables related to cardiovascular health. Specifically, subjects improved on a majority of the variables used to quantify the cardiovascular disease risk profile, demonstrating program efficacy. Subjects, at entry, who were more active, had cardiovascular disease risk profiles indicative of increased cardiovascular health. This supports evidence that habitual exercise contributes to improved cardiovascular health. Subjects who increased exercise duration during the investigation, particularly those who were defined as the most sedentary at entry into the program, demonstrated significant improvements in the twelve risk factors used to quantify the cardiovascular disease risk profile. This supports public health research suggesting that the largest increase to overall population based cardiovascular health may lie in effective programming aimed at the least active segment of our population.

While numerous studies have laid a foundation, additional research is necessary to continue to substantiate the argument that prevention is more proactive, cost-effective, and socially redeeming than conventional medical treatment. As employers continue to examine both the cost-effectiveness and the social efficacy of these programs, further documentation is necessary to continue to strengthen the relationship between health promotion programs, decreased cardiovascular disease, and improved employee health.

REFERENCES

1. Centers for Disease Control and Prevention. *The Promise of Prevention. Reducing the Health and Economic Burden of Chronic Disease.* Atlanta: Department of Health and Human Services, Centers for Disease Control and Prevention, February, 2003.

2. Cerny, F.J. (2001). *Exercise Physiology for Health Care Professionals.* (p. 233). Illinois: Human Kinetics.

3. U.S. Department of Health and Human Services. (1990). *Healthy People 2000 National Health Promotion and Disease Prevention Objectives.* (DHHS Publication No PHS 91-50213). Washington, DC: Government Printing Office (5)392-395.

4. Blair, S. (1996). "Physical inactivity and cardiovascular disease risk in women." *Medicine and Science in Sports and Exercise* 28,9-10.

5. Blair, S. (1995). "Effects of physical activity on cardiovascular disease mortality independent of risk factors. Physical activity and cardiovascular health." NIH Consensus Development Conference Abstract, 77-83.

6. Blair, S. (1994). "Physical activity, fitness, and coronary heart disease." In C. Bouchard, R.J. Shepard, & T. Stephens (Eds.), *Physical Activity, Fitness, and Health: International Proceedings and Consensus Statement* (pp. 579-590). Champaign: Human Kinetics.

7. Paffenberger, R.S., Hyde, R.T., Wing, A.L., Lee, I.M., Jung, D. L., & Kampert, J.B. (1993). "The association of changes in physical activity level and other lifestyle characteristics with mortality among men." *New England Journal of Medicine, 328,* 538-545.

8. Letsch, S.W., Lazenby, H.C., Levit, K.R., & Cowan, C. (1994). "American National Health Expenditures." In P.R. Lee & L.L. Estes (Eds.), *The Nation's Health.* (4th ed., pp. 252-262). Boston: Jones and Bartlett.

9. Centers for Medicare and Medicaid Services. *Health Accounts.* [http://cms.hhs.gov/statistics/nhe/default.asp]. April, 2003.

10. Goetzel, R.Z., Juday, T.R., Ozminkowski, R. (1999). "What's The ROI?" *Association of Worksite Health Promotion Worksite Health.* Summer, 12-21.

CHAPTER TEN

RESOURCES IN HEALTH PROMOTION, EXERCISE, AND NUTRITION

This chapter contains resources for statistical data and research studies, general and supplemental information, and access to additional electronic links in health promotion, exercise, and nutrition. The resources are listed alphabetically

Aerobics and Fitness Association of America
http://www.afaa.com

Agency for Healthcare Research and Quality
www.ahcpr.gov/

American Alliance for Health, Physical Education, Recreation, and Dance (AAHPERD)
http://www.aahperd.org/

American Cancer Society
http://www.cancer.org/

American College of Occupational and Environmental Medicine
http://www.acoem.org

American College of Sports Medicine
http://www.acsm.org/

American Diabetes Association
http://www.diabetes.org/

American Dietetic Association
http://www.eatright.org/

American Heart Association
http://www.americanheart.org

American Institute for Cancer Research
http://www.aicr.org

American Lung Association
http://www.lungusa.org/

American Medical Association
http://www.ama-assn.org/

American Public Health Association
http://www.apha.org

American Society for Nutritional Sciences and American Society for Clinical Nutrition
http://www.asns.org

Anorexia Nervosa and Related Eating Disorders
http://www.anred.com

Arthritis Foundation
http://www.arthritis.org/

Canadian Society for Exercise Physiology
http://www.csep.ca

Center for Nutrition Policy and Promotion
http://www.usda.gov/cnpp/

Centers for Disease Control and Prevention (CDC)
http://www.cdc.gov/

Department of Health and Human Services
http://www.os.dhhs.gov/

Food and Drug Administration (FDA)
http://www.fda.gov

Food and Nutrition Information Center
http://www.nal.usda.gov/fnic/

Food Labeling and Nutrition
http://vm.cfsan.fda.gov/label.html

Food Labeling Information
http://www.nal.usda.gov/fnic/Label/label.html

International Association of Fitness Professionals
http://www.ideafit.com

International Journal of Sports Nutrition
http://www.humankinetics.com/infok/journals/ijsn/intro.htm

Life Clinic
http://www.bloodpressure.com/

Medline (PubMed)
http://www.ncbi.nlm.nih.gov/pubmed/

National Academy of Sciences
http://www.nas.edu/

National Cancer Institute
http://www.nci.nih.gov

National Center for Health Statistics (NCHS)
http://www.cdc.gov/nchs/

National Cholesterol Education Program
http://www.nih.nhlbi.nih.gov/ncep.htm

National Health, Lung, and Blood Institute Information Center
http://www.nhlbi.nih.gov/nhlbi/index.htm

National Institute of Diabetes and Digestive and Kidney Diseases
http://www.niddk.nih.gov/

National Institutes on Aging
http://www.nih.gov/nia/

National Institutes of Health
http://www.nih.gov/

National Mental Health Association
http://www.nmha.org

National Osteoporosis Foundation
http://www.nof.org

National Strength and Conditioning Association (NSCA)
http://www.nsca-lift.org/

North American Association of the Study of Obesity (NAASO)
http://www.naaso.org

New England Journal of Medicine
http://www.nejm.org/

Occupational Health and Safety Administration
http://www.osha.gov

Office of Disease Prevention and Health Promotion
http://odphp.osophs.dhhs.gov/

Quit Net (assistance with smoking cessation)
www.quitnet.org/

State Departments of Public Health
http://www.fsis.usda.gov/ophs/stategov.htm

Sports, Cardiovascular and Wellness Nutritionists (SCAN)
http://www.nutrifit.org

United States and Canada Medical Schools
http://www.mc.vanderbilt.edu/

U.S. Department of Health and Human Services (DHHS)
http://www.os.dhhs.gov

United States Food and Nutrition Information Center
http://www.nalusda.gov/fnic/

United States Sports Academy
http://www.sport.ussa.edu/

Wayne State University Institute of Gerontology
http://www.iog.wayne.edu/govlinks.html

World Health Organization (WHO)
http://www.who.int/

Web MD
http://www.webmd.com

ABOUT THE AUTHOR

Dr. Nellie M. Cyr is a professor at The University of Maine. She teaches courses in the Kinesiology and Physical Education Program within the College of Education and Human Development. Prior to this appointment, Dr. Cyr was the Director of a university based fitness center and employee wellness program. A nationally recognized expert in her discipline, she has authored twenty publications, written and procured almost a million dollars in grants, and has presented cutting edge research at international and national conferences.

A respected leader, Dr. Cyr has served as the President of the Maine State Association for Health, Physical Education, Recreation, and Dance, and as The State of Maine representative to the American College of Sports Medicine.

The youngest of four children, Nellie has earned the notable distinction of being an outstanding athlete. As a teenage prodigy, she entered seven golf tournaments, and won all seven. She is the fourth all-time leading scorer on her high school basketball team, and was a four-year starter and letter winner on both her high school basketball and softball teams.

As a university freshman, Nellie started for the highly acclaimed basketball team, but completed her academic career as a record holder in track and field. She qualified for the NCAA national track and field championship six times, and placed in three national championships. After graduation, Dr. Cyr became a professional and world-class distance runner, and earned the opportunity to compete with the best runners in the world.

She completed her Ph.D. in exercise physiology and epidemiology, where her research focused on the effects of health promotion programming on physiological efficacy.

She is married and currently lives in Maine with her husband Dave.

INDEX

Y